MW01118236

Glowing Reports from Those Who Use Donna Rae's Bodybrushing System:

"I have never known a more valuable health tool, ever!"
—*Jay S., Attorney, Beverly Hills, California*

"Who knew that with just five minutes a day something so simple could turn me into a fanatic about skin care? I have become a Bodybrushing disciple and anyone not doing this is missing out on the amazing feeling of being totally clean."
—*Andrew T., Accountant, Tulsa, Oklahoma*

"Three words. 'Just do this!!!'"
—*David F., Computer Analyst, Seattle, Washington*

"Finally! A miracle that's free! Donna, thank you for showing me how to health myself."
—*Marrisa C., Homemaker, Santa Barbara, California*

"Bodybrushing is an intimate, loving, healthy action I perform daily. Every inch of me is stimulated and invigorated and I literally do GLOW. There is no other way I would start my day!!"

—*Natalie D., M.F.C.C., Spokane, Washington*

"Donna changed the way I think about body care. Now I know how to keep my skin glowing, healthy and working properly."

—*Susan B., Acquisitions Agent, Saratoga, New York*

"Once you start to GLOW, you will never let go. It is the ultimate connection to self-care outside and in. I would advise everyone to get into it."

—*Ashley H., Weight Trainer, Los Angeles, California*

"People should be enlightened about the heightened sensuality and skin sensitivity that evolves with Donna Rae's Bodybrushing system. Touching and feeling with body-brushed skin is a completely different sensation. My partner and I love this new discovery."

—*Allen T. & Patricia T., New York, New York*

"The first thing I noticed after just spending five minutes a day Bodybrushing was that, in less than two weeks, my skin was softer and much less dry. Living in Colorado, and spending a lot of time outside and on horseback, is hard on 50-year-old skin and I've never had much time or interest in long, drawn-out beauty regimens. This is a simple, natural way to look younger. Now I don't think I could start the day without brushing; something would definitely be missing."

—*Victress H., Rancher, Denver, Colorado*

"Since I began skin brushing I have noticed that my skin is softer and less dry. It is relatively easy, painless and inexpensive compared to a salon procedure that would give the same results. The five minutes that it adds to my morning bathroom ritual are easily compensated for by the shorter shower and quicker drying; in fact, my routine now takes half the time it did and it's much more stimulating and effective. Now, instead of singing in the shower, I sing while I'm brushing."

—*Andria B., Opera Singer, Milan, Italy*

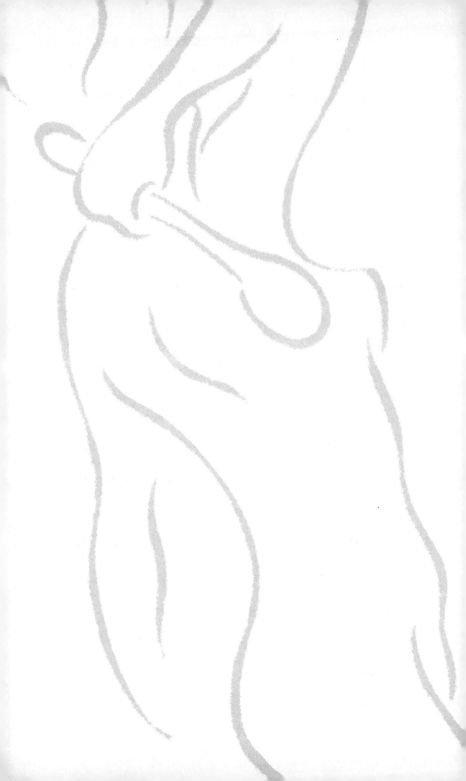

Reveal your GLOW

... brush your body beautiful

Rev

eal your
GLOW

... brush your body beautiful

Donna Rae

EarthTime Publications
Santa Barbara, California

Reveal Your GLOW: Brush Your Body Beautiful by Donna Rae

Published by: EarthTime Publications
1324 State Street, Suite J292
Santa Barbara, California 93101

Edited by: Gail M. Kearns, GMK Editorial Services, Santa Barbara, California

Copyedited by: Barbara Coster, Cross–t.i, Copyediting, Santa Barbara, California

Book and Jacket Design by: Matt Hahn, ThinkDesign, Buellton, California

Cover Photography by: Mony Photography, Santa Barbara, California

Interior photographic illustrations manipulated by Matt Hahn from original black and white photographs by Mony Photography

Line illustrations by Matt Hahn adapted from sketches by Entéra

Printed in the United States of America

Library of Congress Catalog Number
98-92618

ISBN 0-9663286-3-9

Rae, Donna
        Reveal your glow : brush your body beautiful / Donna
    Rae -- 1st ed.
        p. cm
        Includes bibliographical references.
        Preassigned LCCN: 98-92618
        ISBN: 0-9663286-3-9

    1. Skin--Care and hygiene. 2. Beauty, Personal. 3
Mind and body. I. Title

RL85.R34 1998   646 7'26
                                 QBI98-1149

This book

is dedicated

to every person

on the planet

seeking simplicity,

strength and

radiant,

glowing

health.

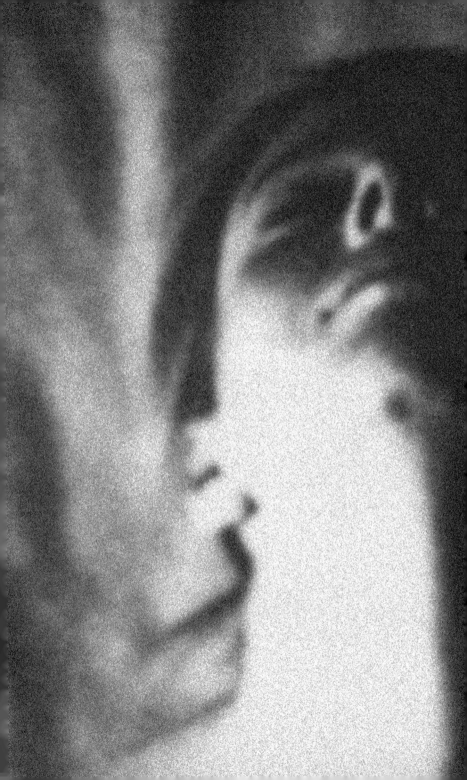

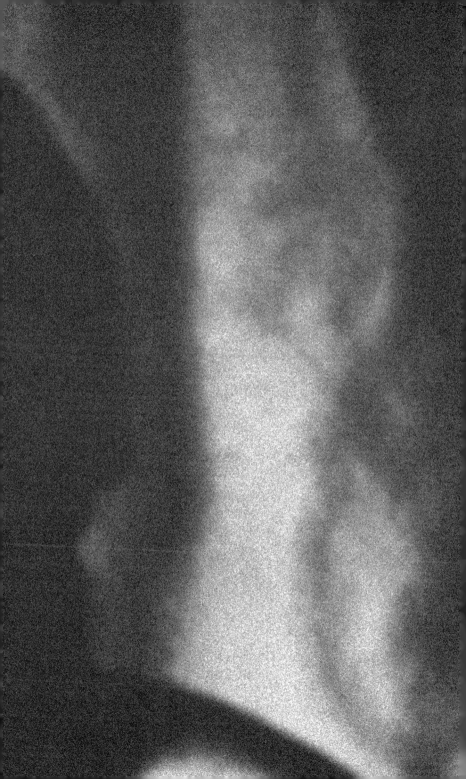

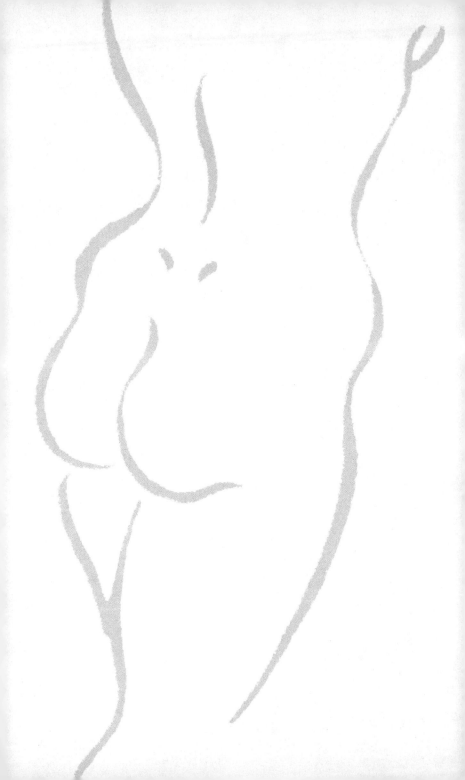

Table of Contents

Acknowledgments

I want to thank the many people who have touched my life
and helped bring this book to fruition.

To Shanti, my angel and soul mate, my pillar. The one person
who gave me the courage to follow my truth.

Gail Kearns, my editor and motivation monitor, you "got it"
from the first moment and made this project "Glow" in print.

Dr. Herb Gravitz, thank you for introducing me to a
whole new language.

My guru, Dan Poynter, the largest self-publishing tornado
to ever hit the Western Hemisphere!

Matt Hahn, artist, designer and creator of beautiful books!!

My beautiful visionary children, Kristal, Tom and Jaclyn, thank
you for believing in me every moment.

*I thank and appreciate the Universe for supplying
all that I needed, and then some,
so that I could give this gift to every one of you!*

Let's Get Glowing!

My passion for helping people introduce a simple and purifying ritual into their daily body care routine resulted in this book. My one wish is that those of you reading this book will become motivated to make Bodybrushing your lifelong companion. I understand that each of you who begins my Bodybrushing program will personalize this experience to suit your own individual lifestyle. Bodybrushing is not new. In fact, it has been a beauty secret of men and women for ages. From Greeks to Romans to Native Americans, this ritual of exfoliation is age-old. I am taking the wisdom of the ancients and turning it into practical application which you can use to Reveal Your Glow.

"Donna Rae is changing the way the world wakes up."

Does that sound crazy? Well, at first, all of my friends thought I was a bit loony. But every last one of them has become a true devotee of my ten-minute, four-step skin care routine. They can't wait to wake up in the morning so they can start brushing for healthier, livelier, glowing skin!!

At one point in my life, I was so overwhelmed with information about skin care that I decided to do nothing at all and see if it worked. I found out that "nothing at all" works okay—for a short while. At least I had less stress to deal with in the amount of work I *thought* it took to have skin like a spa goddess. My only desire was to find THE ONE THING that would get me truly connected to my body—that would get my circulation going, get me a healthier lymphatic system, foster a connection within and maintain radiant, gorgeous skin. Naturally, that one thing had to be really QUICK AND EASY.

It had to be quick and easy because I didn't have time to mess around in the morning. At the time I began my search, I was running two corporations, I had three kids at home and a husband who required at least verbal acknowledgment that I existed in his life. On top of it all, I was studying finance at a local university.

One day, I started reading Dr. Paavo Airola's *Are You Confused?* You have to understand that my library then contained almost every health book that's been in or out of print over the last 20 years. SO, YES, I WAS CONFUSED! However, Dr. Airola was the one man who showed me how to get truly connected to my body. This wonderful nutritionist and naturopathic healer revealed to me a billion dollar health secret—BODYBRUSHING! He called it a secret. I call it a conspiracy on the part of the cosmetics industry, which keeps us in the dark because they might go bankrupt if too many people were to discover this invaluable health secret. Anyway, I took Dr. Airola's advice and designed my own daily routine of Bodybrushing.

The rest of the story goes like this: It worked! Now I look positively alive. My disposition is brighter. I glow! People notice. ("No, I'm not pregnant. I'm just glowing!") Plus, I stumbled upon what has become my passion—and my passion became my profession. I GET MEN AND WOMEN GLOWING!

You might call what I do for a living the most peculiar job in the world! After all, I teach people how to get naked. I don't mean just stripped of clothing and stark buck naked. I mean the absolutely nothing on your body except radiant, glowing skin naked. No chemical-laden soaps, no lotions, no goo—just you.

My friends have since referred me to dozens of other people who cannot believe how simple and rewarding this powerful approach to daily body care can be. To this day, not one of my clients has stopped performing this loving, beautifying ritual on themselves. Many have told me that using this program has made them so much more aware of their bodies and the care of their bodies that they joined a gym, started doing yoga, or began taking vitamins and drinking more water.

In the following chapters, I'm going to give you loads of hot "glow tips" on how to become generally healthier, and how to get glowing and get your blood flowing in less time than it normally takes you to get out the door in the morning. You will learn a completely new and simpler, yet more powerful approach to your daily body care. It's NEW in the sense that you probably haven't done it before. (It's actually a centuries-old concept.) It's SIMPLER because you need very few tools to execute it. It's POWERFUL in its simplicity. I am so happy to be able to share this skin care program with you.

Why am I so passionate about changing the way people wake up in the morning? Read on . . .

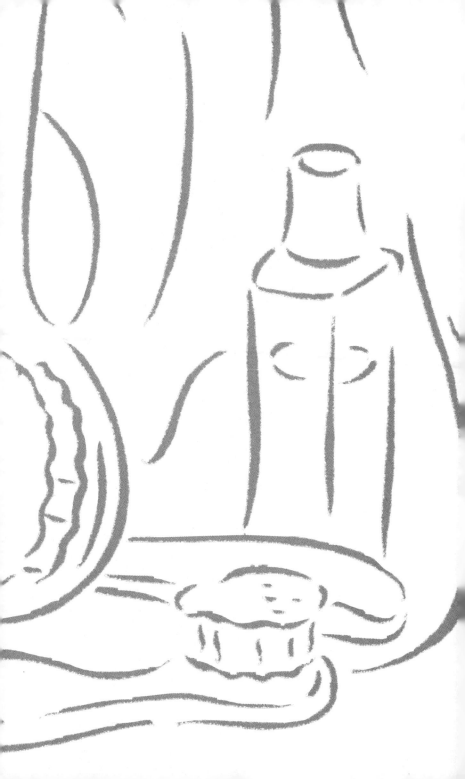

Go for the

glow!

The Glorious Benefits
of Bodybrushing

Imagine you are teetering on the edge of awakening and slumber as you fall into a dream. In this dream you are very, very old, and your body is aching, tired, decrepit and shriveled. Everyone else in this dream seems so alive and vital. You spin around in circles trying to spot someone you know. People rush past you as if you didn't exist. Your life is zooming by. You are on the outside, looking in, trying to connect yourself to something—ANYTHING! "Wait! Wait! Wait for me!!" you scream.

You bolt upright in your bed. You are terrified, drenched in sweat and shaking with fear, anxiety, and a feeling that you are not fully alive and in charge of your own life. Ever had a dream like this? I have. In fact, I used to own that dream, but no longer. That same night, the sad and lonely terror of not having command of my own will ended. I had been slapped in the face with mortality! The reality of how short and sweet life is swept over me like a huge tidal wave—this was the big tsunami!!

From that moment on, I resolved that I would do whatever it takes to never again get lost in the nightmare of not being completely alive and loving every precious moment I have left on this planet. The harsh reality that life is far too short to spend it in poor or even mediocre health finally hit home. Sure, I had always wanted to feel terrific, but I just couldn't get to the place inside me that would commit to taking the steps.

Perhaps some of you reading this book are disconnected and twisted in a downward spiral of bad choices for your outer bodies and inner selves. But you do have a choice. You can have a strong, healthy and vital life or you can remain disconnected and spin off into the void of ill health, self-pity and zero empowerment. Which one will it be?

COME ON, FOLKS, IT'S TIME TO WAKE UP AND START YOUR DAY YELLING AT THE TOP OF YOUR LUNGS, I WANT IT ALL! GIVE IT ALL TO ME NOW!! I WANT TO BE AN ADONIS, A CLEOPATRA, A SPA GODDESS!! I WANT AGELESS BEAUTY!!! I WANT TO GLOW FROM THE OUTSIDE IN AND THE INSIDE OUT!!!

GLOW

૨ ૭

So, you may be wondering, what is GLOW? Glow is the apparent warmth that radiates from within you when you treat yourself with loving kindness. It comes from the practical application of healthy, loving, beautifying rituals on yourself every day. When you treat yourself with caring and kindness, you feel uplifted. This radiates to the outside world. Your luminous glow shines on others. So what are these practical applications? That's what you will learn from this book.

get fit for the journey   Once you become fully aware that you are on this earth for the long haul, you realize there's a lot left to do and you had better have a fine-tuned vehicle to do it in—your body!! Being in good health is absolutely vital, and you might as well look gorgeous in your skin while you're at it. You can get on the path to fine-tuning your body by realizing that you may not be physically, emotionally or spiritually functioning at your optimum best. Do you feel sluggish and depressed? Have you gotten to a place where you aren't feeling good about yourself or enjoying your time here on this planet? Life is too fleeting to miss out on feeling good about yourself. We all need to wake up and perform a loving ritual on ourselves. The tools we need to do this are literally at our fingertips. With my four-step Bodybrushing program, all you need is a body brush, a towel (you don't need soft or fluffy ones either) and some pure plant body oil. And this simple program will put you on a path to discovering your body in a new and exhilarating way. Have you taken a good look at your derriere lately? How about the backs of your upper arms or your elbows? When was the last time you scrutinized your toes, your ankles or your knees? Unless you live in a fun house with lots of mirrors or own a three-way mirror, you probably haven't really looked at many parts of your body at all. But chances are, you have bumps, scaly areas, blotchy patches, and gray, dead skin-cell buildup on some parts of your body and you think it's supposed to be that way. Or maybe you just plain haven't noticed.

mirror mirror on the wall . . .

Taking care of your skin and honoring your body is not about vanity. It's about getting your skin totally healthy, radiant and clean, and getting it to work properly for possibly the first time in your skin's history.

Many people don't understand *how* to care for the largest organ of their bodies—THE SKIN. A lot of people don't even regard their skin as a body organ, when it actually is the most vital part of their entire eliminative system. A whopping majority of humankind has never learned or become aware of a simple, basic approach to skin care that will alter the way they feel about themselves and their bodies. Well, all of this can be changed, and I'm going to show you how. The solution is quick, easy and more stimulating than you ever imagined. You are not only going to have glowing, healthy skin on every single body part—yes, ladies and gents, even your buns will glow—you are going to become hooked on how you accomplish this.

My Bodybrushing program is going to replace the way you take care of yourself right now. It will get you energized, invigorated and glowing externally and internally. AND YOU DON'T HAVE TO WAIT TO SEE THE RESULTS. It's no secret that the four simple steps of this program are designed to give you: #1) super clean radiant skin; #2) super functioning skin; and #3) a super connection to your gorgeous, glowing body in just minutes. You have to experience super functioning skin in order to know what you've been missing.

When you begin Bodybrushing, you will recognize that LESS IS SO, SOOO, SOOOOO MUCH MORE. You will begin to learn about the power of LESS. You will have a tool for life—one that will make you healthy, glowing and connected every day. Why? Because you are going to love how you look and feel from the very first time you perform my Bodybrushing routine, and you simply won't stop doing it. YES! YOU ARE GOING TO CHANGE THE WAY YOU WAKE UP! But that's not all! Your body and the way you think about your total self are going to change right along with it.

"It's just too simple," *electrifying effects* people say. "How can it work so well?" they ask. Some people are true skeptics of my Body-brushing program until they actually per-form it on themselves. At one of my "glow shows" (that's an expression I use for my seminars), I indeed pulled one doubting Thomas up in front of the audience and glowed him right there on the spot. He kept quiet and later thanked me profusely for showing him how to body brush. He hasn't stopped doing it and neither have the numerous clients he sent to me afterward. WHY? Because they have never felt cleaner, more energized or more motivated to care for themselves, and it shows—from their new and radiant skin to their beaming attitudes, these people are all glowing!

One client of mine swears that learning about Bodybrush-ing was invaluable to her. Not only has she saved a substantial amount of time and money by purchasing fewer products, but she feels like she's doing something exceptional for her-self at the start of each day. She avows it is such an uplifting and energizing way to start her morning that she has a better attitude throughout the day about her work and life in gener-al. Then at night, when she has more time to relax, she body brushes away any stress and spends time massaging the much needed oils into her skin. This is pure heaven to her, nurturing herself so simply and beautifully.

Our inherent right as humans is to be contained in a healthy body. In Helen Colton's book *The Gift of Touch,* she tells us that our bodies are constantly trying to stay in balance. This is done mostly through our immune system. If we believe that our body fights for us every minute of every day to maintain some semblance of health, no matter how hard we abuse it, then when we decide to devote ourselves to becoming totally healthy, we have ALL of our being working for us. Our subconscious tells our body, *"We're going to get some help after all. This guy's/gal's stubborn mind is going to connect with us and we're going to get healthy. IT'S ABOUT TIME!! HOW OLD ARE WE NOW?!"* Our entire body chemistry is thrilled when we make this connection.

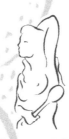

G l o w   T i p
Melt away stress by Bodybrushing for five minutes at the end of each day.

Then what happens? Well, when you begin Bodybrushing—
GET THIS—you will:

~ HAVE DROP-DEAD GORGEOUS SKIN THAT GLOWS
   FROM HEAD TO TOE
~ EXPERIENCE GREAT CIRCULATION—ENOUGH TO
   PUMP BLOOD THROUGH A TEN-FOOT GIANT
~ ACQUIRE A STRONGER IMMUNE SYSTEM BY
   STIMULATING YOUR LYMPHATIC SYSTEM
~ ELIMINATE TOXINS FROM YOUR BODY
~ STOP PREMATURE AGING
~ GROW STRONGER, HEALTHIER NAILS
~ FEEL THE JOY AND POWER OF
   "HEALTHING" YOURSELF
~ SAVE HUNDREDS, MAYBE EVEN THOUSANDS OF
   DOLLARS EVERY YEAR THAT YOU WOULD
   NORMALLY SPEND ON "BEAUTY" PRODUCTS
~ HELP SAVE THE PLANET FROM ABSORBING
   ALL THE WASTE THAT GOES ALONG
   WITH PURCHASE POWER

You are doing your part to save the planet every day when you use my Bodybrushing program. Imagine this! Take six billion people using less water, generating less waste, using less utilities and saving $$$$$—we all get a happier, healthier, wealthier planet.

glowing gracefully

The elderly population is growing rapidly, and by the year 2020 it will be over one-quarter of the world's population. Body-brushing is beneficial for people of all ages.

In fact, I have a dear friend who body brushes her elderly friends and aged family members who can't easily care for themselves. She says it uplifts their spirits. Bodybrushing also brings a high level of care to the elderly who may be incapacitated and need this gentle circulation to their extremities. Another problem we have as we age is that we perspire less. Skin brushing helps to open up the pores and allows the skin to breathe, thus eliminating toxins. Just imagine what could be done for seniors and the incapacitated in nursing homes and elder care centers if Bodybrushing were introduced into their daily care regimen! Bodybrushing is a ritual that goes to the core of one's being. It is a soulful, rejuvenating experience to be enjoyed by all—especially our graceful elders.

GLOW

Anna's Story

My mother, 93 years old, lives in Bavaria. She has skin as silky and fine as a baby's. Naturally, she has wrinkles because she had a very hard life, but the texture of her skin is fresh and young. Why? She gets up at 6 am, opens the window, does two dozen knee bends and then dry brushes her body from top to toe, the movements always toward the heart.

the fact of the matter is ...

In just ten minutes each morning, this simple Bodybrushing routine will get you back on track and get your skin back to work, instead of it being the out-of-commission skin you are used to. The French have a phrase for it—*mal dans sa peau*—which means "to be bad in one's skin." When you start Body-brushing, you will understand how easy it is to give your body what it needs. You will become totally independent from the so-called beauty and cosmetics industry by no longer buying into all the hype. You will know how to get gorgeous, healthy skin naturally. You will become a member of the super healthy skin elite. Quite frankly, it won't be considered elite for long. There's no reason for this system to be known to just a privileged few. The entire planet will be glowing soon.

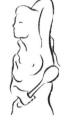

G l o w   T i p
Body brush vigorously in the morning to
energize yourself for the day. It's more
stimulating than a cup of coffee.

My goal is to help you see that your body wants your support, and it will do 95 percent of the work if you just give it permission. You also have to realize you will need to do less, not more. You have to absolutely, unequivocally, trust the simplicity of the Bodybrushing program I am about to outline for you. Simple isn't easy for a lot of people. It means giving up harsh soaps, chemical-laden lotions and long, scalding, acid-mantle-destroying showers. Ultimately, you have to give up thinking that radiant health is something that costs a lot of money and takes even more time. This is NOT the case.

You already have all that you need to get the glowing, healthy, gorgeous body you deserve. Once you begin this Bodybrushing program, you will really begin to understand the power, beauty and freedom of less. Less product, less stress, less waste, less aging. We can all use a little less! And guess what? YOU GET SOOOO MUCH MORE. You are about to own the most powerful body care tool that exists!

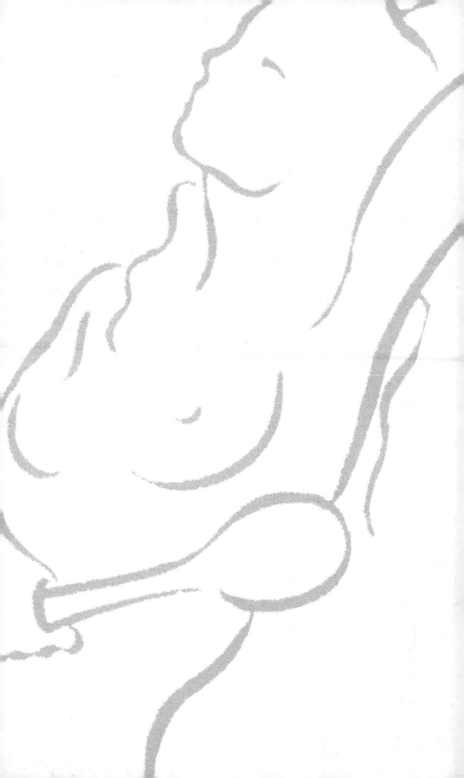

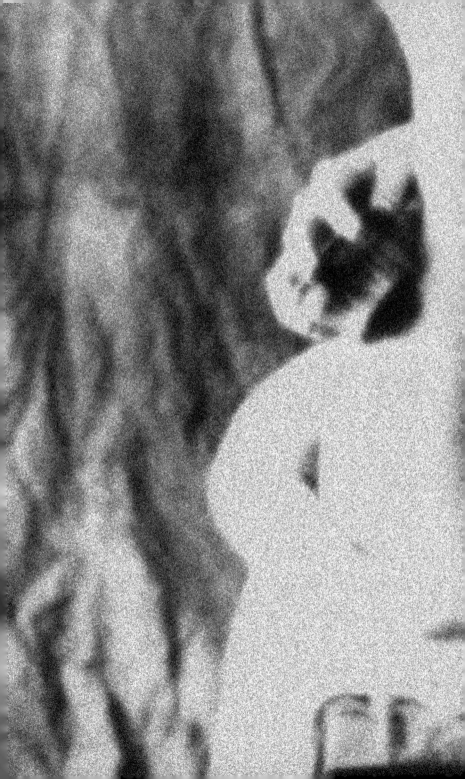

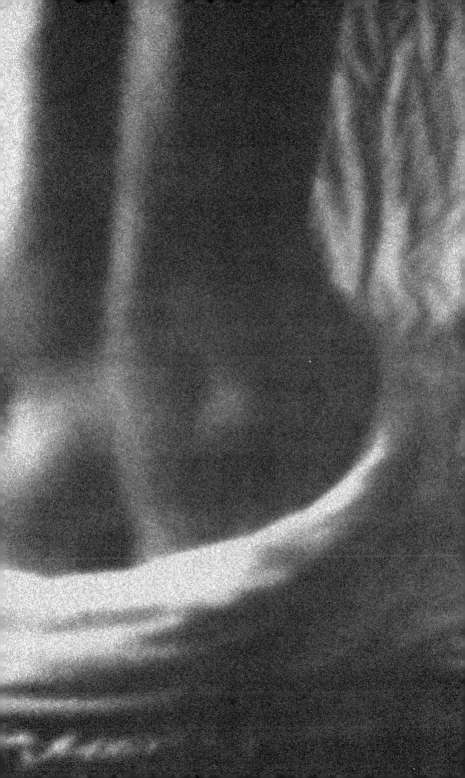

Beautiful

2

lies

What the Cosmetics Industry Won't Tell You

More than 68 percent of Americans are unhappy with some aspect of their physical being. Whether it's their weight, hair, nose, abdomen, whatever—they're continually looking for something out there to fix it. According to Carmen Renee Barry, author of *Is Your Body Trying to Tell You Something?*, "over a million and a half Americans are electing to undergo cosmetic surgery each year." From face-lifts to nose jobs to breast and penile implants, we are a society hell-bent on having the perfect body, the perfect facial features, the perfect pair of breasts and the perfect . . . penis?

Americans also spend over 40 billion dollars a year looking for that one miracle cream, potion or lotion to keep them young looking. I can't believe what the cosmetics companies can sell!! Billion dollar campaigns with dermatologist endorsements. We buy it and, remember, like they said in the magazine ad or on the TV commercial, results could take weeks, so when we use it all up we run out to buy more. Still no results? We try something new. What we NEVER hear is that nothing can stop the natural aging process and nothing should. If any one product does accomplish some kind of miracle aging reversal or halting of the aging process, then why do hundreds of new products with new claims keep appearing on the market every year?

Ever wonder why you keep putting lotion on your hands all day? It's not because you have abnormally dry skin (although that's what we all believe), it's because the lotion draws moisture from your skin. It coats it so heavily that your skin can't do its job, and that job is to keep your acid mantle in place and keep your skin soft, supple and moist. Aubrey Hampton, author of *Natural Organic Hair and Skin Care*, refers to this as the Natural Moisturizing Factor (NMF). NMF is a natural function of the skin. It is a biochemical mixture of oil and water that can be removed or altered by harsh polar solvents, detergent systems and makeup. PEOPLE, WE NEED TO WAKE UP! We buy massive amounts of products in blind faith, thinking that these cosmetics geniuses have our bodies' best interests in mind. HAH!! They bank on our trust.

One of the first things a client of mine noticed when she started Bodybrushing was that she didn't have to apply hand cream to her hands a dozen times a day any longer. And this was right after her first day of using my Bodybrushing program!

stop the insanity Here's the insane cycle. Soaping up in long, hot showers and baths dries out the skin. The cosmetics industry comes to our rescue with zillions of creams, potions and lotions—raspberry, cherry, organic rain flower—lotions for dry skin, sensitive skin, old skin, new skin, whatever the case. It's all chemical-laden goo that supplies a quick fix to our problem. Then it does its real job—it dries us out some more. Then we wash in hot water again, put on more soap scum and cover it up with more Organic Miracle Magic Rain Flower Mist from the Amazon.

pH-balanced products are a bit of a hype. Aubrey Hampton also writes that "a 'pH balanced' product does not protect the skin's 'acid mantle,' and in fact, the substances used to adjust the pH can dry out the skin and hair. . . . The advertising people who thought up the 'pH balanced' slogan forget that the natural pH of the hair and skin is quickly restored after regular washing, so that any alleged value to the 'pH balanced' protection lasts about as long as it takes the products to wash down the drain."

Today's "fountain of youth" cult is a multibillion-dollar industry. We buy products to hide or cover up the signs of aging or we buy creams and lotions we are told will make these signs disappear. Of course, practically NOTHING WORKS and, in fact, in many cases it accelerates the process. Heavy makeup laden with coal tar and petrochemicals will cover up some lines and make us look younger (from afar), but makeup accumulates in all the lines and cracks and blemishes on our face, hence amplifying these areas. Eventually, it will dry out our skin even more and make the lines even more noticeable. In time, all the chemicals and coloring agents in the makeup cause deeper lines, the skin looks older, and we end up using more and more makeup.

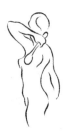

G l o w   T i p
To avoid bursting capillaries, keep the
temperature of your bath or shower water
just slightly above your body temperature.

Jane's Addiction

My dear friend Janie had been hiding behind heavy makeup for over 20 years. She not only USED heavy makeup, she was a cosmetics counter junkie. If it was new and improved and had some secret miracle vanishing wrinkle placenta, she owned it. Eighty dollars an ounce? No problem. That only meant it HAD to be good. Janie was my toughest case ever. She has a natural beauty both inside and out, but she simply could not be seen in public without her makeup. I pleaded with her endlessly just to try my program. Reluctantly, she gave in and started brushing—yes, even her face— as long as it was on one of her days off and she could stay inside so no one would see her without makeup. Over the years, heavy makeup had made Janie's unconcealed facial skin blotchy and pale, mainly because it could not breathe. Nourishment and oxygen were restricted by clogged pores and poor circulation. I made her promise to stop using makeup for two weeks. Well, it took only about three days to see the amazing results. Janie is now completely au naturel. She cleaned out her powder room cabinets of all the useless cosmetics products and got back to basics. She now simply uses a body brush, a towel, and body oil of pure plant oil and vitamins. She wears light powder and lipstick on special occasions, and her boyfriend loves her new look and feel!! She will confess, though, that occasionally she experiences cosmetics counter withdrawal and flashbacks. She still frequents her favorite counters to see all the new products and packaging. And she loves it when people approach her to ask her what products she uses because she really glows. She just smiles, holds up both hands and says, "These and a little TLC. Let me tell you about it . . ." Over the years Janie has referred dozens of clients to me.

Glow Tip
Stop premature aging
of the skin. Give solvents,
soaps and makeup a rest.

the big payoff

The answer really is too simple. You have to take it off. Use fewer products, use a simple and natural approach to body care and watch your skin transform. Let the cosmetics companies suffer—not your skin.

We've been bombarded our whole life with commercials showing relaxing hot baths full of sudsy bubbles, long hot showers followed by an application of some soothing lotion we need to put on our skin for protection. We bought into all this commercial hype and it has destroyed our skin. We prematurely aged ourselves with our bad habits. We jump into a scalding hot shower, destroy our acid mantle, lather on high alkyl sulfate perfumed soaps, then coat ourselves with chemical-laden gooey lotion and call it good for the day. We pay dearly for this with bad skin and thinner pocketbooks. We spend billions of dollars in medical bills on the dozens of different types of skin irritations we suffer from caused by harsh chemicals in the products that we so loyally buy from our favorite cosmetics line.

It's time for you to get the big payoff. So what's the solution? USE NOTHING! ABSOLUTELY NOTHING! YOU NEED TO TAKE IT ALL OFF! Get your skin totally and completely naked for the first time in its life. It's kind of like fasting from food to cleanse your interior, only this time you'll be fasting from products to cleanse your exterior. You need to give your skin a rest. Then get it back to work.

Does the thought of not spending hundreds, even thousands of dollars a year on products that don't work scare you? I'm sure it scares the hell out of the cosmetics industry. Hey, they don't want us to "get it." And it's easy to figure out why. If we find a simple natural solution to perfectly radiant healthy skin, *their* pocketbooks will become considerably thinner. I say, let's turn the tables here, let's get smart, save our money and get totally healthy while we're at it. Let the cosmetics industry sweat it for a change. We don't need their miracle lotion or potion. We need an honest-to-goodness simple, clean approach to getting our bodies back to work for us.

We need to change the way we think or have been programmed to approach our daily body care. We need to think of our daily body care regimen as honoring and loving ourselves. We need to believe that the cosmetics industry doesn't hold our beauty in their bottles—we hold it in our hands. We are the only ones who have the power to make ourselves vibrantly glowing and beautiful. Interested? Read on!

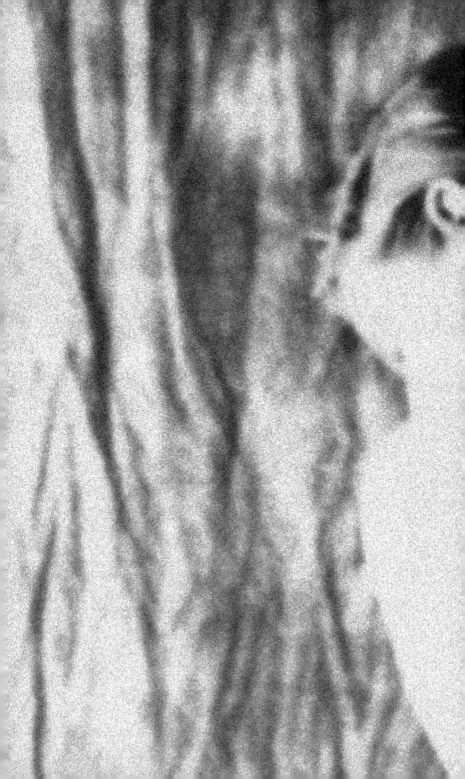

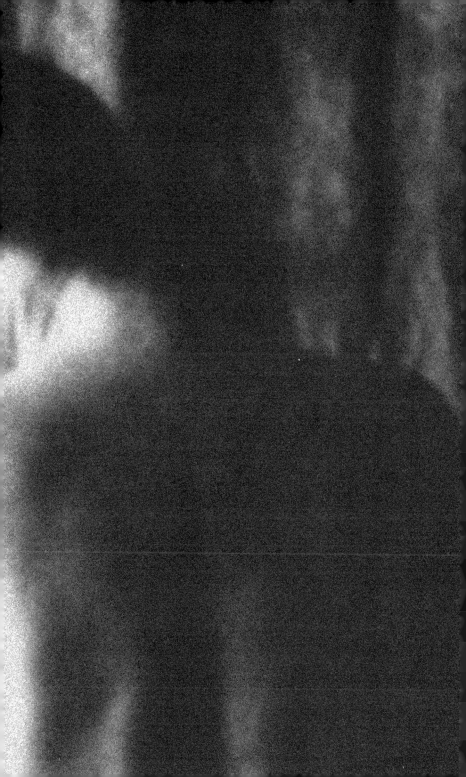

Global

3

glows

I Do It, Swedes Do It, Even Bears Up In the Trees Do It

Lilia empties her basket of ripe avocados into the cleaning basin. She takes the dark green, ripe fruit and scrapes out the fleshy, light green pulp. To this she stirs in her healing salts. Later, when the house is quiet, Lilia fills her tub with warm water. While it is filling, she gently massages the avocado and salt grains into her skin. The salt scrub exfoliates and purifies her skin, and the silky, vitamin rich, oily flesh of the avocado fruit leaves her skin supple and velvety smooth.

Lilia learned this beauty ritual from her Mexican grandmother, who learned it from her mother, who learned it from her mother . . .

GLOW

Undeniably, we all have a lot to learn from the traditions and rituals of our own ancestors. And although there is much cultural diversity all over the world, I still find it fascinating that similar threads appear in many traditions—particularly where cleansing and care of the body is concerned.

What we do know about the healing and beautifying wonders of exfoliation comes to us from various cultures. Exfoliating the outer layer of the skin is done in many different ways in numerous countries. People have known for centuries that exfoliation is necessary for cell renewal, oxygenation and lymphatic stimulation. WHY DID WE LET THIS IMPORTANT HEALTH RITUAL GET AWAY FROM US? IT CERTAINLY ISN'T BECAUSE WE FOUND SOMETHING BETTER TO REPLACE IT WITH, BECAUSE WE DIDN'T.

Native American tribes traditionally practiced exfoliation by using dried corn cobs. The Comanche Indians used sand from the bottom of the Texas rivers to scrub their skin. The Polynesian peoples used seashells to exfoliate. In Finland, people vigorously brushed their bodies with twigs before entering the sauna. Many other cultures used whatever indigenous materials the environment provided: shells, nuts, sand, grains, herbs and plants.

The ancient Greeks and Romans spent hours in their lavish bathhouses rubbing olive oil and salts into their skin and then using a strigil (a long-handled, metal skin scraper) to remove layers of dead skin, sweat and oils.

GLOW

53

The Japanese vigorously brush their skin with loofahs and rough synthetic towels before their traditional hot baths.

Midori's Story

In Japan, as a child, every evening my mother gathered me and my two sisters together before bedtime and vigorously brushed our skin. I remember asking her why she did this. She always replied, "It will keep you from catching a cold." My mother was a doctor so she knew the healthy benefits of physically stimulating the lymph.

Dry skin brushing has been a Scandinavian ritual for thousands of years, not only for its tremendous exfoliating effect on the skin but also for the added boost it gives the immune system by stimulating the circulation of the lymph.

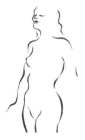

Glow Tip
Bodybrushing is a rite—you can use it to connect with yourself on a deeper level.

Viveka's Story

*I started Bodybrushing in Sweden as early as I can
remember. In school, once a week before class, we
were made to go to the bathhouse. Several classes
would go at one time. I can still recall this kind
of Gothic-looking red brick building. Some older
women were there, dressed in white uniforms.
They were quite intimidating and reminded me
of the stern Russian women who sat minding their
samovars, large metal urns for boiling tea. Only
instead of minding their teapots, they were there
to make sure we brushed properly. If we didn't, we
got a smack on the butt.*

*Inside the bathhouse, there were big tubs filled
with warm water. The uniformed women told us
to get undressed and start brushing. Before we
could get into the tubs, they would inspect our
arms, our backs, our elbows and knees. If they
weren't satisfied, we had to keep on brushing.
It was quite serious. After we finished bathing in
the warm water, boys and girls together jumped
naked into a cold swimming pool nearby. We dried
ourselves off with a rough linen towel, which is
what was available.*

*We did our communal bathing to get clean, of
course, but we also did it because it was in the*

GLOW

♪♪

'40s, after the war years, and the standard of living was not like it is today. Baths in Sweden were not available to everybody. Even soap was rationed. I think our weekly bathing ritual was a way of making sure that no child would feel that they were less important than any other child. In reality, perhaps some children had less, but at least the same opportunities were being made available to everyone.

In the '70s I took my daughter back to Sweden and kids were still going to the bathhouse once a week. So it seems Bodybrushing has become a Swedish tradition in its true sense.

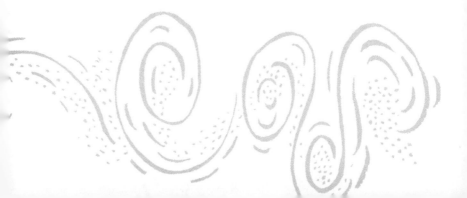

The animal kingdom is way ahead of us when it comes to getting rid of surface dead skin cells. Animals instinctively exfoliate themselves. Bears, deer, horses, cows and many other large thick-skinned animals rub themselves on fences and the scratchy bark of trees. Horses especially know how wonderful a good brushing and rubbing feels.

Why then have so few people heard of Bodybrushing? Have the ancient health and beauty secrets of the ages been kept hidden at exclusive spas only for the well-to-do and privileged to covet?

IT'S TIME FOR THE WORLD TO TAKE BACK ITS TRADITIONS AND RITUALS SURROUNDING THE CLEANSING OF THE BODY. Hey, our ancients had the right idea about skin care. We somehow got too busy, too mechanized, too dependent on dermatologists and other professionals in the Big Beauty Industry, so we gave up the simple, pure rituals of our wise ones.

"get a ritual"

There is something very comforting about rituals, whether they be beauty rituals, religious rituals or holiday rituals with family and loved ones. Rituals foster a connection in yourself to your roots and heritage and to something much larger. Rituals touch you at a deep level that is hard to describe. In *The Secret Language of the Soul* by Jane Hope, she tells us that "rituals both sacred and secular pervade every aspect of our lives, easing us through unfamiliar or difficult situations, and giving structure to our positive experiences of faith." A special ritual can be like the best homecoming you have ever experienced. It remains a constant connection to that place of comfort and familiarity—a place you have come to learn to love and trust.

The Bodybrushing ritual or any other beauty or family ritual becomes a part of you wherever you go. Whatever you do, you take it with you either spiritually or, in the case of Bodybrushing, physically. The brushes and everything else associated with this ritual are totally transportable.

Children instinctively know the importance of rituals. Their constant curiosity about their family history and their yearning for stories about their ancestors make children joyfully accept and desire rituals. Rituals are common among friends as a way of celebrating long and meaningful relationships. Tea parties, luncheons and coffee breaks are rituals people perform in their everyday lives.

Embrace the ritual of Bodybrushing and teach it to your children and your children's children. You can have perfectly working, radiantly clean skin, healthy immune systems, and get tons of circulation and perform a loving ritual on yourself every day. Set the standard for simply beautiful, clean, functioning skin and bring this splendid tradition and ritual into your home.

Later on, I will reveal to you my own ritual—I will give you a bit of my heart and soul. It is a ritual that has become my ULTIMATE connection to the divine power within me. This all started with my daily Bodybrushing program and it has become my ULTIMATE healing and beauty tool.

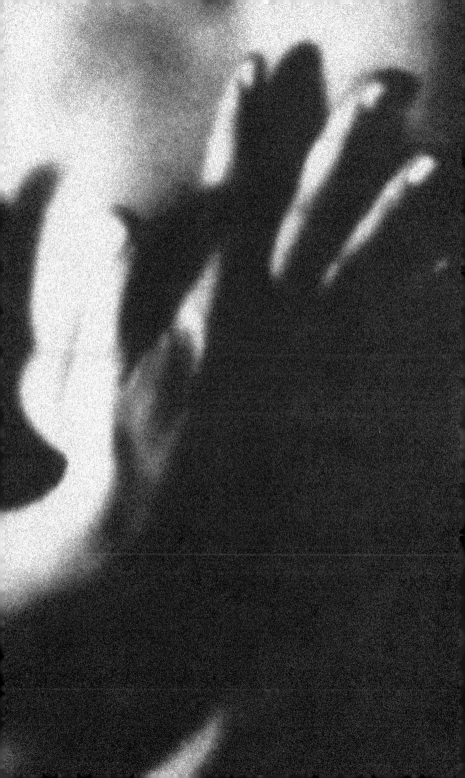

Skin at

work

The Science of Skin

Want to stop premature aging and reduce the risk of degenerative disease? Build a stronger immune system? Get rid of toxins in your body? Sure you do!

HERE'S THE FORMULA:

~ *Dry brush your body every day to improve circulation, which will both prevent waste buildup in your tissues and allow nutrients and oxygen to more freely circulate and nourish your cells.*

HERE'S WHY:

~ *Excess waste buildup in tissues = lack of nourishment and oxygen to cells*

~ *Malnourished cells = slowed down cell generation and impaired cell metabolism*

~ *Impaired cell metabolism and slow cell regeneration = degenerative disease and premature aging*

your skin's job description

(Aside from holding you in and making you look good!)

Aubrey Hampton, again in *Natural Organic Hair and Skin Care*, says, "One square inch of skin contains 650 sweat glands, 78 heat sensors, 13 cold sensors, 1,300 nerve endings that can record pain, 9,500 cells, 19 yards of blood vessels, 78 yards of nerves, 19,500 cells at the end of the nerve fibers and 165 pressure apparatuses for the perception of touch."

The skin is the largest and most important organ of the body. Aside from sensing the elements of hot and cold, recording touch, stimulating the nervous system, and sustaining the network of arteries and lymph ducts that maintain circulation, the skin protects and provides a barrier for our internal organs. It can and does absorb and assimilate nutrients. But its largest and most important role is as an eliminative organ. And that's where YOU and Body-brushing enter the picture. We'll get to that soon.

Glow Tip
Water, water, water—drink it all day long!
It helps to rid your body of toxins.

But first, what does your skin eliminate? Waste—nasty, ugly toxins and lots of them. If your skin is on the job and not clogged and suffocating, it can eliminate up to a pound of toxins a day. Of course, in a perfect world (one with uncontaminated water, oxygen and nutrients, and lots of exercise and stimulation) you wouldn't have to worry about how your skin was functioning.

The skin gets its nourishment from the blood and the lymph as they circulate through the body. The blood gets circulated from the pumping of the heart but the lymph must circulate without this help. That's where Bodybrushing comes in. The lymphatic system is the drainage system for the body tissues. It's where lymphocytes are manufactured, which are made up of white blood cells that produce antibodies that combat infection. Whew!! You can stimulate your own lymphatic system to boost your immune system by dry brushing your skin. It is one of the most powerful ways to cleanse the lymphatic system. Not only do the lymph and blood bring nourishment to the cells, but they also carry waste material away from them. Dry brushing stimulates the release of this waste material from the cells near the surface of the body. Eventually, these toxins, along with their carrier cells, mostly lymphocytes, make their way to the colon.

Our body is an amazing machine that automatically performs self-cleansing and self-protecting functions without any effort on our part. Our body does its cleaning work on autopilot with its specialty team of glands, transportation systems and organs: kidneys, liver, lungs, skin, lymphatic system, alimentary canal, mucus membranes and different cavities. By far, the skin plays a larger role than any of the other organs. Approximately one-third of all impurities are excreted through the skin via thousands of tiny sweat glands (didn't we say our skin eliminates a pound of toxins a day?) that not only regulate our body temperature, but they act like tiny kidneys ready to clean the blood and eliminate these poisons from our bodies.

As I mentioned earlier, the older we get, the less we sweat. Dry skin brushing stimulates our sweat glands and gets our blood circulating to underlying tissues and organs in the body. Our modern, sedentary lifestyle and overuse of antiperspirants also keep us from perspiring enough. What do we get? A backup of toxins and metabolic waste, and this equals premature aging and degenerative disease. Dry brushing opens up the pores and prevents waste buildup in our tissues so our cells can be fed and our organs can function properly.

If all the above seems complicated or too scientific, it's not. The power to get your skin working properly is at your own fingertips. It's easy! With my Bodybrushing routine you can give your skin all the help it needs in ten minutes or less each day. By simply changing the way you look at body care, you'll see how easy it is to get your skin back to work. The super added benefit will be getting connected to healthing yourself at the same time.

We need a holistic approach to our body care—of what is going on inside and outside our bodies so we can take charge and get our skin back to work.

Whether you know it or not, your body comes with its very own operations manual. You mean you haven't read it yet?! Your body tries to communicate with you constantly. It's probably trying to tell you something right now. If any part of your body is dry, rough, pale, puffy, flaccid, blotchy, scaly or otherwise irritated, then you had better pay attention. You are prematurely aging, your cells are not being properly fed and degenerative disease may not be far away.

GLOW

SO COME ON, GRAB AHOLD OF YOURSELF!! TAKE CONTROL OF YOUR BODY AND EXPERIENCE THE AWE-SOME POWER POSITION OF *YOU* HEALTHING YOUR-SELF. THAT MEANS CRACKING THE WHIP A LITTLE AND GETTING YOUR SKIN BACK ON THE JOB. BUT THAT PART IS EASY AND FUN AND EVEN FEELS TERRIFIC.

active skin is in! I know for a fact, based on the astounding billions of dollars spent on ailments and beauty cures, that millions of people suffer the consequences of excessive waste buildup in their tissues. We are prematurely aging and showing the signs of neglect. We just don't understand that the cure can be simple. We need to get our skin back to work.

If your skin is not eliminating properly, breathing properly, absorbing and assimilating nourishing nutrients—then guess what? All of your other organs are put on overtime. You know how it is with any team. When one member lags, all the others have to pick up the slack. Well, when the skin lags, it's no small thing because it plays the biggest part. When the skin is inactive, its pores get choked with copious amounts of dead cells, and uric acid and other impurities remain in the body. This is not good. Your other organs, especially the liver and kidneys, have to work overtime. They labor much harder at the detoxification process and eventually become weakened and diseased.

HERE IS MY ANTI-PREMATURE AGING AND ANTI-DEGENERATIVE
DISEASE FORMULA:

~ SKIN AT WORK = *clean, unclogged, rejuvenated
and properly eliminating organs*

~ SKIN AT WORK = *nourished and oxygenated cells*

~ SKIN AT WORK = *proper cell metabolism
and cell regeneration*

~ SKIN AT WORK = *no premature aging and less
degenerative disease*

*Let's face it—as a society we have evolved into a
sedentary lifestyle. We have autos to transport us and
machines that do what we used to do with physical effort.
As an automated society, we now have to plan our
exercise or activity to get moving and get our blood and
lymph circulating, which brings nutrients
and oxygen to our cells. Getting enough
exercise may be difficult for the many
millions of people who can't get out of
the office or home or for those who
are incapacitated. NOW THERE IS A
SOLUTION. Any person—and that means YOU—can
have all the circulation of a ten-foot giant and beautiful
skin too. Bodybrushing is the ultimate tool. It will definitely give your body more juicy benefits in less time than
any other health tool. There is simply nothing more*

powerful and efficient that you could possibly do to increase your circulation, boost your immune system, unclog your pores, abolish dead skin cells and get absolutely drop-dead gorgeous glowing skin and make the mind-body connection all at the same time in ten minutes or less. Amazing!!

Soon, all your body parts will be working in harmony. Your skin will be back at work and your other organs will be functioning more efficiently. It will show because you will glow!! People will notice that you are managing your body perfectly and they will want to know how. Most glowing people love sharing their management techniques with the world—it's fun!!

NOW LET'S GET STARTED . . .

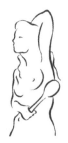

G l o w   T i p
Watch what goes in, it shows on your skin.
Eat lots of crunchy vegetables and fresh fruits
for healthy-looking skin.

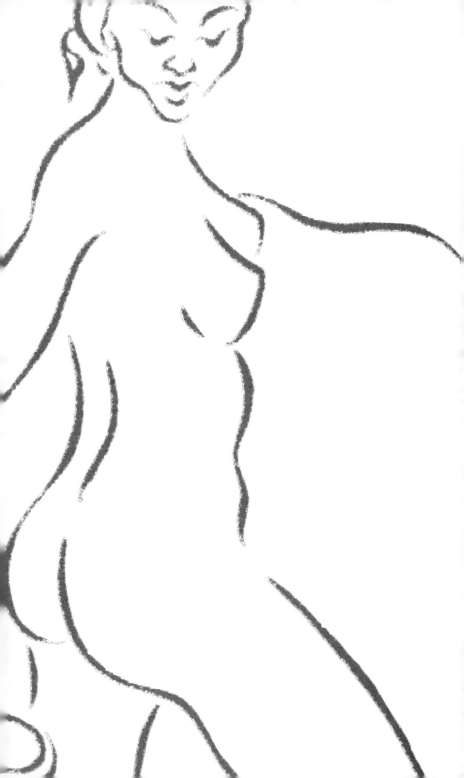

Plugged

in

Getting Connected to "Healthing" Yourself

First of all, in order to get plugged in to this chapter, I want to introduce you to the meaning of "healthing" yourself. That's a term I use a lot. You see, I believe that health is an action word. Good health is using knowledge, action and commitment to maintain a vital state of being no matter what condition you find yourself in.

You cannot separate Bodybrushing from acts of kindness and love toward yourself—and making a body-mind connection. Now, some of you may be saying to yourselves, "Oh no, here she goes with that California crunchy granola stuff." The reason I bring this up AT ALL is that when I told a friend who lives back East that I had devised this amazing Bodybrushing program, she replied, "Sounds very California to me. All that eccentric stuff you get into out there." Well, let me assure you, getting connected is nothing more than doing something good for yourself, committing yourself to a healthy lifestyle, and possessing a great daily vitality. Little did my friend know that Bodybrushing began over centuries ago on another continent—and pretty soon Bodybrushing will become a common morning ritual for folks in Idaho, Sydney, Nigeria, and Burns, Wyoming.

Somehow, many people have the idea that loving oneself and taking good care of one's body is a self-absorbed and self-centered thing to do. I say that self-love is having self-respect, high self-esteem and a healthy self-image—amour propre, *as the French would say. We must deeply and in every way love ourselves. It is essential to our overall health. How do we do this? We have to apply things to our lives that help us get to the place of self-love, for example, how we eat, how we exercise, how we notice our feelings. We begin by gathering knowledge, by finding programs or tools that fit our lifestyle.*

Make the commitment to give yourself all the love and, hence, health you possibly can. I believe the first step on the journey to self-love is desire, wanting the best for yourself, recognizing your internal need for balance, and then making the commitment to give yourself the highest level of health, beauty and wellness within your power. When you know what you want, that's 90 percent of the journey. Getting what you want is mechanical. For this you need the tools, tools you can use daily that will help you maintain a high level of self-honor and self-love. As I've said many times before, life is precious and fleeting, and the only way we can completely appreciate the magnitude of this beautiful gift of life is through love—and most importantly self-love.

G l o w   T i p
Body brush and you are performing
an act of self-love.

Cynthia's Story

*I am very blessed with an abundant life. I can go
to expensive spas and get massage and exotic
body treatments whenever I care to. Many people
do not know such luxuries. Donna's program offers
a solution. She's bringing the elite spa treatments
such as massage and dry brushing home to become
a common household term. Our bathrooms should
be our personal shrine to celebrate the pure joy of
beautifying and touching ourselves. Applying our
own Bodybrushing ritual and manipulating exotic
oils into our skin daily should become second
nature to the masses. Goodness, if the whole world
adored and cared for themselves in this way, it
might even help to bring about world peace!!*

Caring for oneself is where we could all learn something by looking at women (and men, too, I suspect) in other countries and from other cultures around the world. Men and women especially in traditional cultures cultivate their elegance and beauty as they cultivate other aspects of their overall happiness and well-being. They pay attention to their bodies not out of some fear of aging or for purely superficial reasons, but out of a loving attitude toward themselves and as a means to bringing together the mind and body.

In *The Art of the Bath*, authors Sara Slavin and Karl Petzke write about bathing in Japan. They say that "in Japan, bathing has always been an act that transcends its utility. For the Japanese the process of bathing is a ceremony, a ritual that takes the bather to the spirit by way of the body. Whether bathing communally or alone, the Japanese bather washes before getting into the bath. Soaping up, rubbing down, and using a small bucket to rinse, one not only washes away the world's dust, but prepares the mind for a deeper cleansing— the bath that follows. The warm bath water calms both body and mind, bringing about a languid ease, and daily concerns fall away. . . ." For centuries, all over the world, men and women have used the bath as a ritual to transcend the purely physical realm to a place of calm and serenity—a way of coming home to oneself.

If you live a life of wisdom and grace, people are drawn to you. You radiate and give forth a genuine warmth toward others. If you do not honor and love yourself, it shows. The whole world sees it. As a matter of fact, you may have an unloved body. Is your body pale and flaccid? Is your body overweight, over-worked, tired and worn? These are all signs of neglect, which you can turn around with love for yourself.

When you make the commitment to finally get connected, your whole world changes. The act of performing a loving, healthy ritual on your body every day transforms you even if only for the few moments you are performing the act. Those moments uplift your soul. You feel blissful and satisfied that you accomplished a loving act. You begin to seek other avenues of self-love and exploration. The gap between your mind and body grows smaller, and soon you begin to realize it is the ultimate journey. When the path to self-discovery, self-expression and self-love is familiar to you, you will GLOW and your light will shine on others. Total and complete self-love really is the ultimate goal you can attain here on this planet.

survival mode

Many people are alienated from their bodies and they don't even know it. By this I mean they are living in "survival mode." Survival mode is the whirlpool in our subconscious mind that spins our thoughts downward to places of procrastination and self-disgust. Everyone suffers some degree of survival mode syndrome, even if they have the perfect job and are able to pay the bills on time. They may be the ones who are saying things like, "If only I could lose these extra ten pounds, but I don't have the time to exercise," or "Maybe if I had the time, I could find the right mate," or what about, "I'd eat and sleep better if I weren't so stressed out all the time."

You are in survival mode when you are just hanging on and trying to get from one day to the next. You are not being creative or living your life's dream.

The mental energy used up each day by people existing in survival mode constitutes one-half to two-thirds of their waking hours. Multiply these numbers by the millions of people existing in survival mode and you'll discover that the amount of energy wasted in this unproductive, self-flagellating state of mind is staggering.

You might be wondering, *So what does Bodybrushing have to do with all of this?* Well, I truly feel that Bodybrushing is the missing link to total self-care. This simple program provides you with new habits that connect you to every single aspect of your physical well-being and to your mental and spiritual well-being. You see, once you start Bodybrushing, you begin a metamorphosis. You notice how gorgeous your skin is getting, how soft and supple it feels. You notice more color in your skin and you feel more energized and invigorated. You want to share this with your friends, especially your mate if you have one. (If you don't have one, believe me, you'll start thinking more about getting one soon!)

Nicky's Story

After just two days of brushing my skin I began to notice a finer quality about it. It was smoother, softer and more alive feeling. My circulation seemed to have restarted after years of dormancy. Now I brush to wake myself up in the morning; it's more effective than a strong cup of coffee. Next will be the ultimate test—to have someone else feel my beautiful new skin!

When you start my Bodybrushing program, you also begin connecting with other people in a more positive way. You are no longer dwelling in a place of survival mode about self-care. You are excited about the positive changes you are making in your daily routine, and you may even notice that you are more concerned about your diet. Perhaps, you think, it's time to find a simple approach to eating, one that you can adapt to your daily routine and still enjoy. Maybe you start taking walks and smelling the roses along the way. Then you decide to go to the next level of fitness and look for other ways to exercise. You join a gym or start taking yoga classes. Now you are living more in the present and loving how you feel. This is a fairly common scenario when people start to employ my Bodybrushing system. They really begin to feel the simplicity and power that comes with healthing themselves.

But let me tell you a story about Ellie, who takes it even one step further. When I met Ellie, she was living a life of quiet anxiety—alone in a huge home with three children, an alcoholic, verbally abusive husband and a mentally unstable father-in-law. Like so many people, Ellie was absorbed in her day-to-day survival issues, but she refused to succumb totally to her unhealthy environment. In Ellie's mind there was always a way out. She just wasn't sure what it was yet.

When I first started my Bodybrushing program, Ellie was one of the first people I approached. I thought she needed a little nurturing and would enjoy the benefits of Bodybrushing. Back then, even for me, Bodybrushing was simply a mechanical beauty aid to help reveal utterly gorgeous skin. A totally NOW sort of thing. I had no idea what the universe had in store for my Bodybrushing system, nor did I know how powerful a tool it would be to getting connected and finding a path to self-love. Of all the people who started this program, Ellie taught me the most profound lesson. I'm immensely thankful to her for showing me how the simple act of cleansing the skin can be transformed into an act of self-love.

What Ellie revealed to me changed the way I think of self-care. To this day, she calls Bodybrushing her own private path to self-discovery. She has healed herself, and not just because of my program. Granted, Bodybrushing was the impetus that got her to pay attention to her body and to signs of neglect, but she has since gotten professional help to heal some deep internal scars. She never gave up seeking a dynamic life against seemingly outrageous odds. Today, she is awake and vitally alive, loving life, loving herself, and finally giving love. After all, until you love yourself, you cannot fully and unconditionally begin to TOUCH the lives of others with love.

skin is emotional

Many of us are starving, not from malnutrition, but from lack of touch. We don't get touched enough and we're afraid to touch ourselves. We are literally cut off, disconnected from our own bodies. Our fast-paced lives make it easy to ignore our bodies, especially our skin. And often, even the most blatant calls for attention such as disease, pain and discomfort are ignored. We need to be aware just how important a role our skin plays in our entire well-being. John Heinerman, author of *Encyclopedia of Anti-Aging Remedies*, states that "the skin, more than any other part of the body, tells the world how you feel about yourself, mentally, emotionally and physically."

TOUCHING IS NOURISHMENT FOR THE SKIN. TOUCHING, RUBBING AND MANIPULATING YOUR SKIN WILL TRANSFORM IT INTO A HEALTHY, VITAL ORGAN. IF YOU ARE NOT NURTURING YOUR SKIN BY STIMULATING TOUCH, IT IS NOT AS HEALTHY AS IT SHOULD BE—PERIOD. Until you start Bodybrushing, your skin may look and act like it's starving. It may be pale and dry, with bumps and gray buildup on your knuckles, elbows and knees. You may have hangnails and poor cuticles. There are millions of people walking around today who don't know that their skin has a job to do, and if they literally don't get their hands on themselves and get their skin back to work, it will show!!

Touch helps our bodies maintain homeostasis, the harmonic interaction of all of our body parts—electrical energy, blood, bones, hormones, enzymes and muscle tissue. The body is constantly striving to maintain a homeostatic balance. As we learn how our system works, we understand how important a role touching plays in our overall health.

Our bodies have more than five million receptors for touch. This is a lot of opportunity for healing ourselves. In Helen Colton's book *The Gift of Touch,* she writes, "Touch stimulates the production of chemicals in the brain and these feed our blood, muscle tissue, nerve cells, glands, hormones and organs. Deprived of touch to stimulate these chemicals, we may be as starved as if we were deprived of food."

the ultimate connection

One of my clients is a massage and acupressure therapist. She discussed with me the Chinese approach to power centers or *chi*. When I told her that many of my Bodybrushing clients hadn't gotten a cold for over a year, let alone the flu or allergies, she explained that, according to Chinese medicine, the skin and lungs are closely linked because the lungs supply the energy to the lymph and the lymph stimulates the immune system. Hence, if you are giving your skin stimulus and loving touch every day, it is highly positive to your immune system. Isn't it amazing how everything connects?

When you begin Bodybrushing, you'll be astonished at all the connections you'll be making as well as the number of outstanding issues being resolved such as:

~ HOW TO GET RADIANT SKIN
~ HOW TO LOVINGLY TOUCH YOURSELF EVERY DAY
~ HOW TO GET MORE CIRCULATION GOING THROUGHOUT YOUR BODY
~ HOW TO STIMULATE THE LYMPHATIC SYSTEM, AS DESCRIBED ABOVE
~ HOW TO CHANGE THE WAY YOU LOOK AND FEEL
~ HOW TO MAKE THE BODY-MIND CONNECTION

G l o w   T i p
Give yourself ten minutes
of quiet time each day.

A woman in her seventh month of pregnancy asked me if I thought Bodybrushing would help with the circulation in her legs. She was getting severe cramps every night and it was disturbing her sleep. "Well, it can't hurt," I told her. "Let's get you on this program." It worked. Her cramps disappeared. She even stopped brushing once just to see if it really was the program that was working. She got a cramp the very first night. It got rid of any doubts in her mind. However, she did call me about a month after she started Bodybrushing and expressed some anxiety. Apparently her husband loved her new supple skin so much that he couldn't keep himself from touching her. "Boy, what timing," she said. "I'm ready to deliver this baby and he's all over me. He does love the ritual, though, and he even helps to brush the parts of my body where my tummy gets in the way."

Glow Tip
Use touch to heal. It is the most important of all our senses in the healing process.

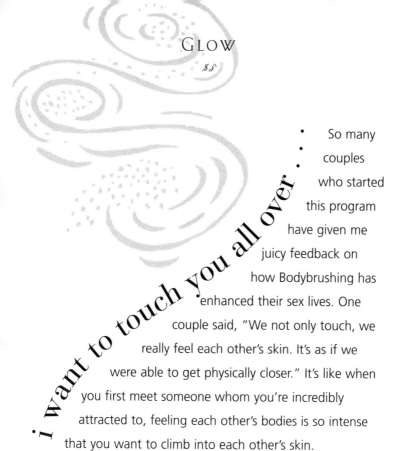

i want to touch you all over

So many
couples
who started
this program
have given me
juicy feedback on
how Bodybrushing has
enhanced their sex lives. One
couple said, "We not only touch, we
really feel each other's skin. It's as if we
were able to get physically closer." It's like when
you first meet someone whom you're incredibly
attracted to, feeling each other's bodies is so intense
that you want to climb into each other's skin.

Another couple said, "My partner won't stop touching my
soft new skin." Still another said, "I want my husband to rub
his hands all over me now. It's odd, but I love the way my skin
feels and I want my mate to feel me too." That's what Bodybrushing can do for you and your partner. It can bring
back that lovin' feeling.

Naturally, you will have your own particular feelings about
this program. Use this as an opportunity to encourage your
partner to join in this loving ritual. Enrolling your mate to simply
brush your body can be a stimulating experience.

The

6

f u l l

monty

Feeling Comfortable about Getting Naked, Really Naked!

She prances through the house on her tiptoes, joyfully singing her favorite tune and waving a silky scarf like a graceful ballerina without a tutu—stark naked. That's Rachel, a friend's nine-year-old, free-spirited daughter. Her mother endlessly urges her to put something on—anything—so Rachel prances back through the room with a hat on, or gloves. She thinks she's very funny. She lives in a busy household with people coming and going constantly, and her mother is worried that some people may not appreciate a free-spirited, creative, uninhibited little soul running around naked. In truth, most of us have forgotten how wonderful it feels just to get naked and let our skin breathe unencumbered by any clothing.

Our skin is a breathing, living, vital organ. It requires oxygen to maintain proper cell regeneration. Constrict any part of the body with the pressure of a belt that's too tight or even a collar and watch the discoloration. We need to let our skin out more often. Let it come out and play. Prance around for a while in our birthday suit and feel how exhilarating it can be. Act like my friend's nine-year-old daughter, a prepubescent spirit exploring the beauty and wonder of bare skin—touching, feeling and playing innocently—and completely free to expose our beautiful bare self to the elements.

naked rites

Air bathing—ever heard of it? Air bathing is getting naked and letting your skin breathe as you perform some sort of exercise. It could be stretching out in the morning, doing push-ups or simply meditating. People in Sweden have been air bathing for hundreds of years. The more I learn about different cultures and how they care for themselves, the more determined I am to transplant other enriching traditions and rituals to my life here and now. We lost souls here in North America, and perhaps in many other countries, need to adapt some of these age-old health secrets and call them our own. Or at least begin to originate our own rites of passage.

Here are a few suggestions:

~ CREATE YOUR OWN AIR BATHING RITUAL. GET NAKED
  IN FRONT OF AN OPEN WINDOW OR A MIRROR, GET
  YOUR BODY MOVING AND LET YOUR SKIN BREATHE.
  SWING YOUR ARMS AROUND AND MOVE YOUR HIPS.

~ WEAR PAJAMAS ONLY BEFORE BEDTIME BUT MAKE
  THEM TABOO UNDER THE COVERS. KEEP THEM OFF
  WHILE YOU ARE SLEEPING AND LET YOUR SKIN HAVE
  ITS FREEDOM.

~ DO SOME YOGA OR MILD STRETCHING EXERCISES
  WHEN NAKED. IT'S EXTREMELY EXHILARATING.

~ BODY BRUSH EVERY SINGLE DAY FOR THE REST OF
  YOUR LIFE. WHILE YOU MANIPULATE THE OILS INTO
  YOUR SKIN, GET IN TOUCH WITH YOUR ENERGY
  CENTERS, ALSO KNOWN AS CHAKRAS.

Peter Kelder, author of *Ancient Secret of the Fountain of Youth*,
wrote about the importance of reactivating your energy centers
on a daily basis.

Robin's Wish
I would be ecstatic if one of the things my children remembered about me was how well I cared for myself. I would love it if my health habits got passed down to them and to their children.

naked, naked, naked . . .

Ever Seen a Grown Man (or Woman) Naked?

Really, what is the big deal here? Why can some of us face our naked bodies and others shudder at the thought? I'm not going to get philosophical or psychological here, BUT . . . What is, IS, and there is nothing I can say here that will change any PSY-CHOLOGICAL issues that may be preventing some of us from looking at our own naked bodies and exploring and gathering information available on the exterior of our bodies—our skin. And just because some of us can get naked and like to prance around sharing our glory with the universe doesn't mean we are any healthier or happier than those who cannot go there. It just means we can get naked. So what?! What I am hoping for is some useful nakedness, if that's possible. Getting naked for our physical and emotional well-being and getting to know our body and read what it is trying to tell us. Getting naked to let our skin breathe unencumbered and really feeling comfortable, clean and pure in our own skin.

1580 - Queen Elizabeth dyed her hair red, plucked her eyebrows and whitened her face. She was the first English queen to see herself in a clear glass mirror. She banned mirrors from court as she aged.

Once you've made the choice to vibrate on the level of super health, you need to understand there are two different types of nakedness: the no-clothes-birthday-suit naked and the absolutely-nothing-on-your-skin-stripped-clean-of-chemical-laden-goo naked. You want to achieve both. In order to get totally super healthy clean skin, you need to body brush every day. This will bring you the ultimate in naked pure healthy skin. You will then own the ultimate health and beauty tool.

GLOW

92

Lynn, a client who suffers from obesity, called me and wanted a private consultation. She asked that I show her my program and pleaded that I demonstrate it on myself first so she could see how it was done. That was okay with me, no problem. She was shy, I thought, and that's fine. She made the commitment to give it a try for two weeks and thanked me. I didn't hear from Lynn for almost a month. Finally, I called her on the phone. It turned out that Lynn was very uncomfortable with the intimacy of my program and she didn't want to admit to me that she couldn't do it. When she got naked and began the brushing, she felt so uncomfortable that she put the brushes away, put the kit up in her cupboard, and she hadn't touched it since the first attempt. "I can't stand to look at myself," she finally blurted out. "I see what I've become and it is so disgusting that I actually HATE YOUR PROGRAM!! It makes me focus on what I'm trying to hide from myself and the world." WOW!!!I was dumbfounded.

At first I took Lynn's pronouncement personally—hey, I'm sensitive too—but then I realized her reaction was good. My Bodybrushing program really is a path to self-discovery. Whether it be love or disgust, we must know where we stand with ourselves. No one had ever expressed their self-disgust to me so bluntly. I was determined to help Lynn, though, so I asked her to let me show her another way—a more subtle approach to getting to know her body. First, I went out and purchased an XXL cotton robe. Then I set up a time when we could meet in the privacy of Lynn's home. When the time came, I asked her to put on the cotton robe and to begin the steps of my Bodybrushing program with her eyes closed—feeling her way through the steps simply by touch. I explained that this would help her in many ways but I emphasized the purely biological benefits—getting rid of toxins, feeling more circulation in her body immediately, and feeling the increase in energy and vitality. I did not talk about the sensual aspect of Bodybrushing—how beautiful she would feel, how soft and supple her skin would be, how wonderful it would be to touch and manipulate her skin, or that she could even begin to love taking care of herself. Lynn wasn't ready to approach that part of herself. She could not imagine anything beautiful about herself and therefore would not believe anything, especially that her own hands could transform her into what she imagined only in her dreams.

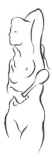

G l o w   T i p
Get naked and read your skin. Red blotchy
patches, grayness and bumps signify ill ease.

So, I forbade her to look. I told her she could even perform the steps in a dark closet if that's what it took. From that day on, Lynn began Bodybrushing every day. I don't know if she resorted to doing it in a dark closet or not. It wouldn't matter if she did. The point is, she is out of the closet now and she won't stop Bodybrushing—ever. Now, early each morning in front of her mirror, Lynn brushes her body, rinses, buffs her body dry, and rubs exotic oils into her glowing, well-loved body.

The benefits of getting naked are, of course, circulation, stimulation, super clean exfoliation, oxygenation, invigoration and a lot of the other -ations. But really, the biggest benefit is one of self-realization. You get to see what you created—all of it.

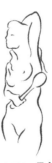

G l o w   T i p
Get naked and let your skin breathe in the
sunlight and fresh air. It feels good.

look at your precious body and choose

Take
action if you
feel you need to
change any or all of
what you have
created. By this I mean:

You can lovingly accept yourself
just as you are and recognize that
you may not be ready for change . . . OR
You can lovingly accept that you are a healthy,
beautiful and wise soul constantly seeking a
higher level of health, beauty and knowledge with
every breath, every moment.

I hope you choose the latter path and begin breathing,
brushing, toweling, rubbing oil into your body and prancing
naked around your room—joyful and happy that you CHOOSE
TO VIBRATE IN SUPER HEALTH.

know thyself The power of getting connected to your body and knowing how to care for it can be transforming. Being able to look at your skin as a barometer for your inner and outer health is relatively easy. Stress, ill health and imbalances show up in many different forms—some are much more obvious than others—but once you're in tune, you begin to notice even the most subtle signs your body gives you.

Do you have bumps, scales or spider veins? There are so many signs of ill health and disease that can be caught or prevented by just being in touch, and I mean literally in touch, every day with your skin—all of it. Are you overweight, underweight, malnourished?

LOOK AT YOUR NAKED SELF. You created everything you see. I know this can be a harsh reality for some of us, but it's also very exciting because you can re-create your body every day that you are alive. You can make it all that you want it to be. Do you desire total health? You can have it. You can re-create YOU every moment of every day. You can choose good health!

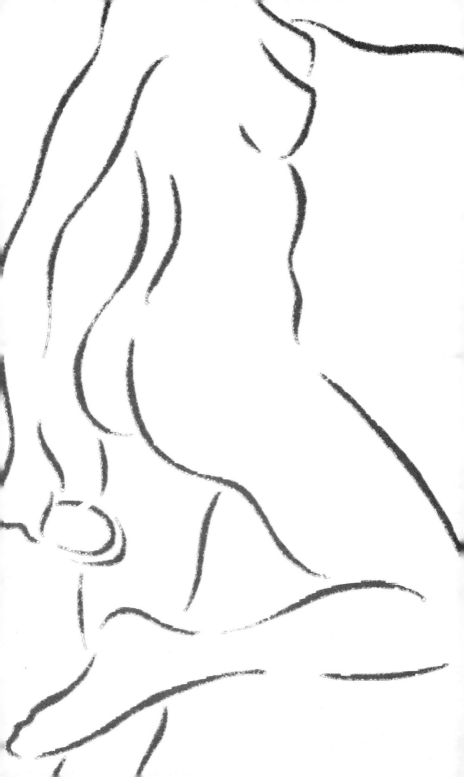

The great

7

o i l

scare

Debunking the Myth about Applying Oil to Your Body

Cleopatra, Aphrodite, Helen of Troy, King Tut and Jesus. They all benefitted from the beauty, health and anti-aging properties in pure plant oils. "Oil free" was a term unheard of in those days. Entire countries were ransomed for a few ounces of exotic oils . . . well, maybe not entire countries, but at least a few small villages.

WE HAVE BEEN MISLED, FOLKS! Contrary to popular beliefs, oils are essential to your skin's health and beauty. John Heinerman, in *Encyclopedia of Anti-Aging Remedies,* writes about how essential fatty acids or EFAs are vital to the health of the skin. Our bodies cannot produce them. They must come from the diet or supplements. He says, "The two EFAs are omega 3 (alpha-linolenic acid) and omega 6 (linoleic acid). Four of the very best sources for such omega-3 fatty acids are: cod liver oil (1 tbsp daily), flaxseed oil (2 teaspoons daily), olive oil (1 tbsp daily), and evening primrose oil (4 capsules daily)."

We have come to believe that oils clog the skin and cause skin eruptions. Creamy chemical-laden products do just that. But a body that is lacking the proper oils also has the side effects of dry, parched, aging skin. Take all the fats and oils out of your diet and out of your skin care products and you will go from being a plump juicy grape to a dried-up old raisin long before your time.

7500 B.C. - Egyptian shepherds and hunters in the Nile valley used oil crushed from castor beans to protect their skin from the sun.

Dan, a dear friend and Bodybrushing disciple, loves the brushing part of my program. He says it just makes him feel so much cleaner than he's ever felt before. One day, as we were driving to Los Angeles for one of Dan's lectures at the Learning Annex, I took a look at his hands and noticed that they were dried out and wrinkled. "Dan, you're not using the oils I blended for you, are you?" I exclaimed. He gave me a really sheepish look and said, "No, I don't like oil. I've only used lotion on my skin. Oil makes me feel sort of greasy." "Get over it," I chided. "You haven't even tried it yet, have you?" I had him feel the skin on my arms and legs, which are not at all greasy. "Look," I said, "I use oil every day and my skin is soft, velvety and supple.

It isn't greasy because the oils are immediately absorbed. They don't stay on the surface and clog up my skin. Dan, you have to at least try it before you say no." By the end of our one-sided debate, I think I had him convinced that he wouldn't turn into a greasy french fry if he used a little of my special blend of oils on his body after showering.

Toss out all your preconceived notions about oil being greasy! As I've said before, oils are not only essential, they are vital to your skin's health and beauty. When used in the proper quantity and applied in the right way, oils are not messy. Your skin absorbs them immediately. Use them daily, but use the right kind. The following list is a guide to the best oils for the outside of your skin and for the inside so you can continue to generate healthy, glowing cells. They are also perfectly suitable for consumption. Try them on your favorite salad.

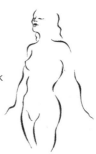

Glow Tip
Oils heal. Pour some in your bath and soak
in warm, luxurious splendor to
Vivaldi and candlelight.

200 - The Greek physician Galen mixed water, beeswax and olive oil into a cream. On the face the water evaporated, cooling the skin. Modern cold cream is virtually the same mixture.

AVOCADO OIL is a wonderful, non-irritating oil that I use as a base for all my blended body oils. Each ounce is packed with many active ingredients like vitamin A (20,000 I.U.), vitamin D (40,000 I.U.) and vitamin E (300 I.U.).

CARROT OIL has tons of vitamins and is a super skin food. It is also non-irritating, so you can use it topically.

EVENING PRIMROSE OIL is a super-powered, super beauty oil packed with essential fatty acids. Use it topically and take it internally.

OLIVE OIL contains essential fatty acids and is a good, non-irritating base oil. It is one of the best oils you can take internally.

WHEAT GERM OIL is packed with vitamin E and essential fatty acids, and is also a good, non-irritating base oil.

SUNFLOWER OIL also has lots of essential fatty acids and is virtually non-irritating.

do it yourself—blending your own oils

The beauty of blending your own oils is that you get to customize them to your own special needs and liking. You'll find that blending your own oils is also simple, fun and liberating. You'll want to use a six-ounce jar for blending your oils. The vitamins you'll use come in gel caps. You can stick them with a pin or snip them with a pair of scissors and squeeze the vitamins into the jar. Put the lid on and shake vigorously.

Below is the formula I blend for my clients.

THE GLOW OIL RECIPE

~ POUR FOUR OUNCES OF A BASE OIL
  (usually avocado because of its rich, active ingredients)
  INTO A SIX-OUNCE CONTAINER OR JAR.

~ ADD 500 MG EACH OF VITAMINS A, D AND E.

~ AS A FINISHING TOUCH, ADD 2,000 MG OF
  EVENING PRIMROSE OIL.

You can purchase all the above oils and vitamins at your local health food store. (See Resources in the Appendix.)

Try apricot kernel oil as an even lighter base and add some

of your own essentials oils, like lavender, rose or jasmine for a flowery scent if you like. Make sure you include the vitamins listed in the above recipe.

You don't need to use much of any body oil—just a few drops on each part of your body. It is light and absorbs easily into your skin. It leaves absolutely no oily or greasy residue. I have noticed—and many of my clients have mentioned—that the more your body gets used to the brushing and oils, the more you absorb. I use quite a bit more oil now than I did when I first started my daily Bodybrushing program over a decade ago.

1700 - Powder rooms became fashionable in Europe and America because men and women powdered their hair, wigs and faces. In bed, women put oiled cloths on their foreheads and wore gloves to prevent wrinkles.

Gina's Story

*I bumped into Gina at the corner General
Nutrition Center (GNC). She was staring blankly
at the vitamin section of the shelf. I had to reach
around her to get the vitamins I was looking for.
Then I moved along to the evening primrose and
shoved several boxes of it into my basket. All the
while, Gina was standing there in a daze. She
was like I used to be. Very confused!! There is too
much stuff and we don't know what works or how
to make it work. Too much wonderful information
just makes us short circuit. If every product is the
best, then why are there so many different bests
and which is the best for any one person? It drives
people crazy!! Anyway, I could see that Gina
needed rescuing. I went up to her and held out
my hands. I asked her to feel them. I do this often.
Most people are shocked or they think I'm nuts,
but we all need a jolt and most people are
responsive once they see I'm harmless. I explained
how oils and a simple Bodybrushing program
would give her hands and her entire body a
beautiful, supple glow—and I told her that about
a hundred other amazing healthy things would
happen to her too. Sometimes I feel sort of like a
crusader running around saving people. I*

promptly educated Gina on how to begin her own Bodybrushing regimen. Gina is no longer dazed and confused in the GNC store. She learned that simple, pure plant oils and vitamins can give her skin a soft, supple and vital glow. Now I imagine Gina walking up to completely dazed strangers in the vitamin aisle at GNC, and with confidence she holds out her hands and shows them how young and gorgeous her skin looks. She picks up a bottle of evening primrose and begins, "Just blend these vitamins with some avocado oil and . . ."

The most consistently dramatic visual results of my Bodybrushing program—and I truly believe the oils and brushing make the biggest difference here—are on the hands and feet, elbows, ankles and knees of daily body brushers. Your extremities literally are transformed into amazingly pretty, glowing, manicured and young-looking body parts. Even your nails and cuticles benefit.

Julie's Story

I had weak and brittle nails all my life. I could never get them to grow and I always suffered from unsightly hangnails. I was into Donna's Body-brushing program for about a month when I made an appointment with the manicurist whom I had been seeing for years. As she dipped my fingers into the warm water, she exclaimed, "Julie, you have nails. I've never seen your cuticles and nails so healthy before."
Of course, I had to divulge my secret new fetish!!!

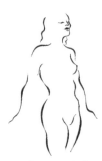

When you body brush, your whole body will change, but it is evident how thirsty your neglected extremities are and how starved they are for attention. The immediate, dramatic, beautifying results of pure plant oils was humorously summed up by one of my clients when she wrote, "I had exceedingly rough elbows, knees and ankles, which at 36 had taken on the ashen look of a weathered elephant. . . . The dryness which has plagued me all my life has disappeared. My skin feels softer and is more supple to the touch."

Glow Tip

Rub oils on lavishly before bedtime and
wrap yourself in a cotton robe, sip chamomile
tea and fall asleep while reading your
favorite soulful book.

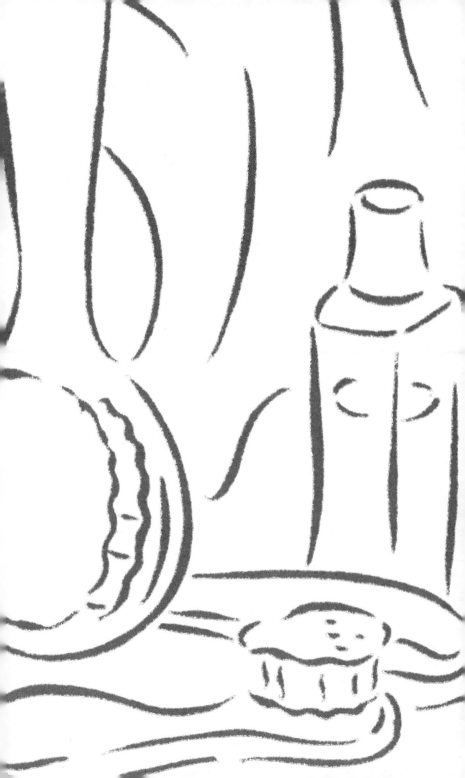

The big

chill

Confessions of a Shower Addict

I don't know about you but for me showering is very close to heaven. That first burst of warm water running over my groggy morning limbs feels so tingly and wonderful. I shower in the morning to wake up. I bathe at night to relax. I shower during a cold spell to get warm. I shower when I'm stressed. I shower to celebrate a change in the weather. I imagine the closest on earth we ever get to the womb is in the warm, enveloping waters of the bath or shower. Too Freudian for you? Maybe, but I've often thought I could save a lot of money and replace my therapist with shower and bath sessions. My best ideas come to me in the shower. Granted, I may sometimes get a bit carried away with showering and bathing. But I absolutely, unequivocally, adore my shower and bath time. Slipping into the velvety warm water of a tub laced with herbal oils, with soft candlelight glowing, sipping herbal tea and listening to a Brahms violin concerto has become a ritual in my life. OOOHHH, what bliss!

GLOW

For a long while, I also got carried away in the soap depart-
ment. I owned soap for every part of my body—in every color,
shape and size—AND from two to twenty bucks a bar. Years
ago, when I started compiling research for my Bodybrushing
program, I read a few things that distressed me a whole lot.
Things about water temperature and the length of the bath—
AND SOAP. I went into COMPLETE DENIAL about some of the
information I was digging up. I put it away! I wouldn't include
it. It couldn't be true and it probably wouldn't be useful to
anyone on this planet! Certainly no one would want to know
about these findings anyway.

You see, not only did I love bathing and showering, I
loved lathering up in hot, hot water. And what I learned
through my research was not supporting me in this. In fact,
almost everything I read was telling me to lower the water
temperature and not to use soap, that I was damaging my
skin and causing premature aging by using harsh soaps and
excessively hot water. I didn't like this. Not one bit!! My one
obsession involved soap and hot water, so please!!

I just couldn't throw out my $18 bar of soap! I just couldn't
turn the water temperature down and not soak for two hours
in the tub. Then I read somewhere that I should give myself a
cold splash of water right before I got out of the shower or
before stepping out of the bath. Not on your life!! Never!! Not
me. I wanted to be wild and free with my shower and forget
all this so-called health-heeding advice.

My rebellious attitude didn't last long. The research I had gathered started haunting me. Every time I got into the shower, I would step out as red as a lobster from the steaming hot water. I began to wonder how many surface capillaries I had burst and how high I had raised my body temperature. I knew that skin cells age more quickly as the temperature of the body rises, especially when the body's attempt to cool itself is thwarted by irregularly long hot showers.

Needless to say, I began paying more attention to what I was doing to my skin. Soap was drying it out and destroying its protective acid mantle. The acid mantle is the protective layer of fatty acids from the sebum. Soap was clogging my pores and leaving a filmy layer of chemicals and synthetic perfumes on my skin. More than that, my skin was absorbing this rubbish.

GET THIS! THE BIG CHILL!! A FEW SECONDS OF COLD WATER GIVES YOU THESE BENEFITS:

~ ACCELERATES BLOOD FLOW

~ RAISES BLOOD PRESSURE

~ HELPS FLUSH THE ELIMINATIVE ORGANS AFTER THEIR NIGHT'S WORK

~ HELPS REGULATE THE BODY'S TEMPERATURE BY CONTRACTING AND DILATING THE CUTANEOUS VASCULAR SYSTEM

~ GIVES TONE TO THE ENTIRE NERVOUS MECHANISM OF YOUR BODY

~ KEEPS NORMAL FUNCTION OF THE SKIN AT PAR, THUS AIDS AND RELIEVES OTHER ELIMINATIVE ORGANS OF THE BODY

(Source: *JAMA, Journal of the American Medical Association*)

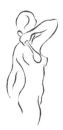

G l o w   T i p
Give yourself one cold spurt of water at
the end of your daily shower to help regulate
your body temperature.

I have to admit, the older I get, the more I appreciate the healthy tips from the anti-aging masters. Following are some tips on soap and water and how you can use them wisely. Or not! It took me a while to appreciate the rejuvenating and stimulating effects of cold water spurts. I know that many of my clients still shudder at even the thought of using cold water.

Bodybrushing eliminates the need for soap. I know this is tough to swallow, but it's true. Use only a light glycerin soap (I recommend Body Shine's Unsoap or Kiehls Baby Soap) on your private parts. Bodybrushing will get you cleaner than any soap ever will, I assure you. You will notice a dramatic difference in the level of your skin's moisture when you stop using soap.

Enjoy a soak in your tub for 20 minutes or less. Any longer will dry out your skin. Keep the temperature to warm (slightly above body temperature. If your skin turns a vivid pink, the water is too hot). Extremely hot water will burst your surface capillaries and destroy the skin's protective acid mantle. A high increase in body temperature speeds up the aging process of cells. Warm and cold bursts of water are good for your circulation, and your body's immune system benefits when exposed to both warm and cold temperatures back to back.

Water is the ultimate healing tool. When used wisely, it can transform your tired, aching body into a rejuvenated, refreshed body ready to take on the world.

Cold showers and no soap? What is this? Some sort of masochistic beauty torture? Those are words from some of my clients. Look, you don't have to employ these methods. You can do what you've always done and get the same results that you have always gotten. Or you can save hundreds, even thousands of dollars, save your skin, unclog your pores, have better circulation, less dryness, no irritations, and get back your own internal beautifying skin protection system (your acid mantle). Just turn down the temperature of your bath or shower water and use less soap. You can do it!! It's like detoxing. You have to start slowly so you don't send your system into shock. You may go through some withdrawals and scald yourself a few more times. Tossing out all that perfumed soap may be too much for you at first. Break into it slowly. But remember, the facts may haunt you too as you continue to destroy your skin's acid mantle by slathering on all that chemical-laden goo and killing perfectly healthy skin cells before their time. What's worse, you have the facts now. You are doing this fully conscious of the long-term consequences. But go ahead and enjoy yourself. Enjoy your scalding bath while it lasts. You'll eventually give it up in the end—just as I did.

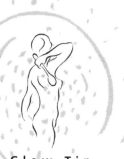

G l o w T i p
Bodybrushing eliminates the need for soaps and lotions and you save money too.

Twenty years down the road, when your skin still looks youthful and radiant, you will be living proof of the power and beauty of less—less soap, less lotion, less chemical-laden goo!!!

Getting

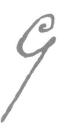

started

The Tools You Need

The tools you need to get started with my Bodybrushing program are surprisingly simple. You may already have some of them at your disposal in your own home, and the rest can be purchased easily at your local health food store or ordered from the back of this book.

Donna Rae's Story

I used to be a bathroom sleuth. Whenever I was invited to someone's home for dinner or any other occasion, I would make my obligatory trip to the bathroom and conduct my secret poll. I would check out the products and supplies on the counter tops. Always to my complete horror I would see the most obscene things that people used in their regular body care routines—

like perfumed soaps, lotions and creams loaded with chemicals and tons of other gunk to clog up the pores. Pale as a ghost, palms sweating, I would return to the hosts and festivities, and sometimes even sidle up to one of them and try to touch their skin. I must confess, I felt a little like Inspector Clouseau. Secretly I would say to myself, If only I could give them a clue about the awesome benefits of Bodybrushing, it could solve all of their skin nightmares.

Your bathroom should be a reflection of how you care for yourself. One attractive bottle of body oil, a couple of beautiful wooden brushes and a clean cotton towel on the counter. Can this be it?? Could this simplicity really work?? You bet it does— and immediately too!

Before I consult with a new client, I insist that he or she commit to my Bodybrushing program for a minimum of two weeks. When I arrive at the client's home, I enter with a stack of towels under my arm, a couple of brushes, and enough body oil to get the client through 14 days on the program. Then I start clearing out their bathroom shelves and drawers of all the products they don't need. I tell them that if after two weeks they want these chemical-laden products back, I will gladly comply. In the meantime, I put all the lotions, creams and miracle whatevers into a bag labeled with the client's name and take it with me when I leave. Why? Because the idea is to get the space for taking care of their body as clean, pure and simple as possible, and those products unfortunately are not helping them. They are cluttering up their space and clogging up their pores.

After two weeks, I come back and we celebrate with a bon voyage party where clients get to toss out more of the stuff they don't need any longer. It's such an exhilarating feeling to know that all you've ever needed to have perfectly healthy skin was less than you could ever imagine. I love to go to my clients' bathrooms now. When I see their precious little crunchy towels hanging on the rack, the basket of brushes and the single beautiful bottle of pure plant oil on their counter, I get this triumphant feeling of joy. These people really understand the power, beauty and freedom of less!

super "health" yourself Naturally, the ultimate motivation for Bodybrushing is your will and desire. You must want super health for yourself. And the very first place to begin this journey is with the exterior purification of the body—what you do every day as a matter of habit—your morning shower or bath.

~ Your HANDS are the first tool and they are an integral part of all four steps of my Bodybrushing program. Your hands hold the brushes; they work with the towel in the buffing step; they manipulate the pure plant body oils into your skin.

~ The actual BRUSHES are the second tool you'll need (see list of resources in the Appendix). You will want to purchase a long-handled, stiff vegetable bristle brush for most parts of your body and a short-handled, softer vegetable bristle brush for the chest and neck area. You can also work with this softer brush on other parts of your body if your skin is too sensitive for the stiffer brush. But eventually you will be using the stiff brush all over except for your face. There are small round brushes available on the market that you can buy for your face.

~ The third tool you'll need are a few inexpensive, coarse
TERRY CLOTH "BUFFERI" TOWELS. I found a place
that sells them wholesale and I love them (see the Appendix).
You will only use one a day. That's all!! So three towels would
be enough to get you through to clothes washing time.

*Save all of your soft, fluffy, plush towels for the
in-laws. They won't know the difference and
will think you're being gracious. If you
have totally cool in-laws, share the health
secrets of Bodybrushing with them and
take them out to buy their own tools.*

~ Finally, the fourth tool of ultra importance is the PURE
PLANT BODY OIL you will be using to replace all of your
lotions, soaps and chemical-laden goos. I have included recipes
for these oils as well as resources for excellent, already blended
body oils. You will find the recipes in chapter 7 and the
resources in the Appendix.

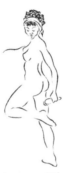

That's it, folks!!! Your hands, a towel, a brush and some body oil. These simple tools and the four steps outlined in this book will give you quantum leaps in the health and beauty of your skin. And I promise—
YOU WILL REVEAL YOUR GLOW!

Glow Tip

Less is more. You need only a brush,
a towel and a small bottle of oil in your daily
body care routine.

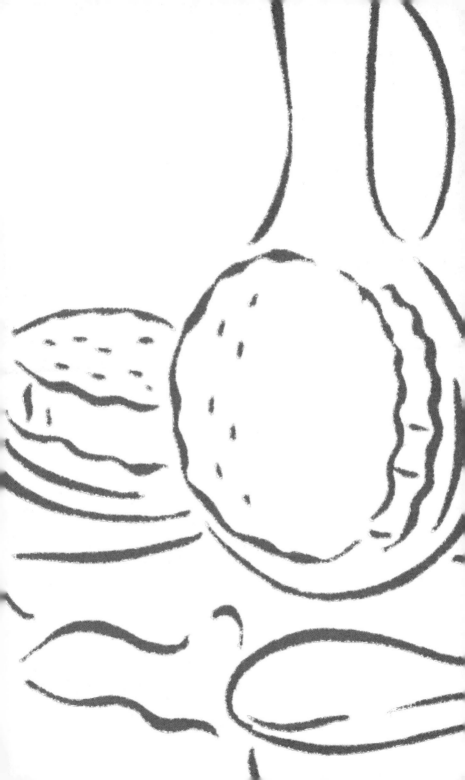

Reveal

Utterly

B e a u t i f u l

skin

The Four-Step **RUBS** Routine: Brush, Rinse, Buff, Rub

A dmit it! You skipped the first nine chapters of this book because you wanted to get started at once with my four-step Body-brushing routine, didn't you? Well, if you did, BRAVO! That means you're already committed to "super healthing" yourself. You can always go back and read the other chapters at your leisure.

My Bodybrushing program has four steps: Brush, Rinse, Buff and Rub (apply oil). It is designed to be used around your morning routine in the bathroom and it should take no more than ten minutes of your precious time. SO WITHOUT FURTHER ADO, LET'S GET GLOWING!

STEP #1—THE BRUSH

First, you will exfoliate your skin. You can do this outside or inside the shower stall or tub. But don't turn on the water just yet. You will be gently brushing each part of your body several times, overlapping the strokes slightly to cover the entire area being worked on.

So, go on . . .

GET NAKED AND GRAB YOUR LONG-HANDLED BRUSH.

~ START WITH TINY CIRCULAR STROKES ON YOUR TOES AND WORK YOUR WAY UP YOUR FEET TO YOUR ANKLES AND CALVES, ALWAYS STROKING AWAY FROM THE EXTREMITIES TOWARD THE HEART.

~ STOP AT YOUR KNEES AND BRUSH THEM VIGOROUSLY, ESPECIALLY IF THEY ARE DRY AND SCALY.

~ THEN GO TO YOUR THIGHS, AND REACH AROUND AND VIGOROUSLY BRUSH YOUR BUTTOCKS.

~ BRUSH ACROSS YOUR LOWER ABDOMEN, STOMACH AND LOWER CHEST AREA.

~ REMEMBER TO BRUSH UP THE SIDES OF YOUR RIBS
AND UNDER YOUR ARMPITS. THIS IS A GREAT PLACE
TO STIMULATE THE LYMPH.

~ REACH FOR YOUR BACK, AND BRUSH AS FAR
AS YOU CAN.

~ FINISH WITH YOUR ARMS AND EACH HAND.
BRUSH VIGOROUSLY ON THE BACKS OF YOUR
HANDS AND FINGERTIPS.

~ NOW GRASP YOUR SOFTER SHORT-HANDLED BRUSH
AND BRUSH LIGHTLY ON YOUR UPPER CHEST AND
NECK AREA, BOTH FRONT AND BACK.

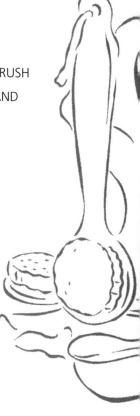

~ IF YOU CHOOSE, YOU CAN BRUSH YOUR FACE TOO.
BUT GO VERY GENTLY HERE. USE THE SMALL
ROUND BRUSH DESIGNED FOR THIS JOB. FACE
BRUSHING CAN EVEN OUT THE TONE OF YOUR
FACIAL SKIN AND LEAVE IT WITH A WARM,
HEALTHY GLOW.

~ EVEN YOUR EARS WILL APPRECIATE THE SOFT
STIMULATION OF A BRUSH, OR USE YOUR OWN
FINGERS TO LIGHTLY MASSAGE YOUR
EARS AND SCALP.

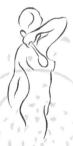

Glow Tip
Add to the pleasure of your Bodybrushing
routine. Choose some music to glow by.

STEP #2—THE RINSE

Whether you opt for a claw-foot tub or a shower stall, you need to think of your bath routine a little differently at this point. Think of your shower as a rinse. THE CARDINAL RULE IS TO KEEP YOUR BATH OR SHOWER SHORT AND THE WATER TEPID. *Remember, hot water strips the natural oils from your skin and bursts surface capillaries.* Besides, you've already "cleaned" your skin by brushing it. You are now just rinsing off the dead skin cells.

~ JUMP INTO A LUKEWARM SHOWER OR BATH. IF YOU MUST USE SOAP, MAKE IT A GLYCERIN SOAP, BODY SHINE'S UNSOAP OR KIEHLS BABY SOAP.

~ IF IT'S TIME, OR YOU THINK YOU'RE GOING TO HAVE A BAD HAIR DAY, WASH YOUR HAIR WITH YOUR FAVORITE SHAMPOO.

~ GIVE YOURSELF A BLAST OF COLD WATER AT THE END OF YOUR SHOWER OR BATH. SPIN AROUND TO GET THE FULL BENEFIT. IF IT HELPS, YOU CAN CURSE AND SCREAM DURING THIS PART OF THE RINSE.

~ JUMP OUT! YOU'RE FINISHED WITH THE RINSE.

STEP #3—THE BUFF

Notice how your blood has rushed to the surface of your already glowing, rosy skin to warm you up. You feel cozy even before you begin toweling off. Now you are going to experience the ultimate luxury of buffing your body dry. Zombie-like, most of us just step out of the tub without thinking about our towel as a tool. Toweling is yet another perfect opportunity to give your body more circulation and stimulation. You will use the same toes-to-heart technique as you did with your brushing.

~ GET A GOOD GRIP ON YOUR COARSE TOWEL AND BUFF IN A CIRCULAR MOTION. START WITH YOUR FEET AND DON'T FORGET THOSE TOES. BUFF EACH TOE, PUSHING BACK THE CUTICLES AS YOU RUB.

~ BUFF UP TO THE ANKLES AND CALVES.

~ BUFF UP TO YOUR THIGHS, BUTTOCKS AND STOMACH.

~ BUFF YOUR ELBOWS AND ARMS.

~ CURL YOUR FINGERS AND BUFF THEM VIGOROUSLY BACK AND FORTH ON THE TOWEL. AS I SAID, THIS HELPS TO STRENGTHEN YOUR NAILS AND CONDITION YOUR CUTICLES.

~ MOVE TO YOUR CHEST AND NECK AND END WITH A LIGHT CIRCULAR MOTION ON YOUR FACE.

VOILA! YOU HAVE JUST PERFORMED MAGIC ON YOUR BODY AND SOON THIS AMAZING TOWELING TECHNIQUE WILL BECOME SECOND NATURE TO YOU.

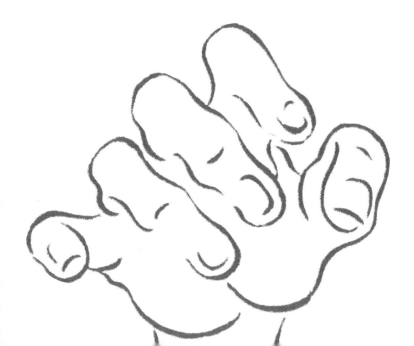

STEP #4—THE RUB (APPLY OIL)

Now your body is perfectly primed to absorb the vitamin-packed oil. Your skin is now ready for its drink of pure plant oil packed with vitamins A, D and E—the best moisturizer you can use. THAT'S IT! THAT'S ALL YOU NEED. NOTHING MORE, NADA. SO LET'S **R**EVEAL **U**TTERLY **B**EAUTIFUL **S**KIN NOW . . .

~ APPLY A DIME-SIZED AMOUNT OF OIL TO YOUR PALM (A LITTLE GOES A LONG WAY), THEN RUB YOUR PALMS TOGETHER TO OBTAIN AN EVEN APPLICATION.

~ USING THE SAME TECHNIQUE AS YOU DID WITH BRUSHING AND BUFFING, MASSAGE THE OIL INTO

EVERY PART OF YOUR BODY, STARTING WITH YOUR TOES AND WORKING YOUR WAY UP TO YOUR CALVES, THIGHS, ETC.

~ USE YOUR FINGERS TO WORK DOWN INTO THE MUSCLES
OF YOUR LEGS, ARMS, ABDOMEN AND BUTTOCKS. YOU
SHOULD BE RUBBING YOUR BODY SO VIGOROUSLY THAT
YOUR HEART RATE INCREASES AND YOUR BREATHING
BECOMES DEEPER.

~ WHEN YOU GET TO YOUR FACE, SPRITZ A LITTLE WATER
ON IT BEFORE YOU LIGHTLY DAB ON THE OIL.

~ ENLIST THE HELP OF A LOVED ONE TO APPLY OIL TO
YOUR BACK OR BE SATISFIED THAT YOUR BODY IS
NOW 95 PERCENT COMPLETELY
GLOWING!!

Health,

mind and

body

The Divine Power
Within Your Body

Earlier in this book I told you I would reveal to you my own personal self-healthing ritual. Here it is! YOU CAN OWN IT TOO! Some of you will love how this works and others may find it a bit odd. I hope everyone who reads this book will at least try the following ritual while they body brush. It is the perfect way to connect with your powerful energy centers every day.

Holistic healing means healing the whole complete person (i.e., body, soul, personality and spirit) in relationship to the outer world. I believe we should take every opportunity to perform holistic healing rituals on our body as an alternative to modern medicine and as a preventative measure. And what better opportunity to do this than during our everyday body cleansing routine.

The human body contains seven major energy centers or chakras, as the Hindus call them. The Sanskrit word "chakra" means "wheel"—a wheel of energy within the body. These chakras are situated at various levels on the spinal column, which is the conduit for all energies going into or coming out of the body. The chakras are like power points on the spine. They are also each related to an endocrine gland, which secretes hormones. These hormones regulate every major function of the body. Diet, environment, stress and emotional health all affect our hormones.

There are many wonderful books that explain these chakras in detail. Caroline Myss's *Anatomy of the Spirit* is one of my favorites. Basically, all that we are is energy. All that we do, say, think and feel is recorded in our cells and reflected in our physical and emotional selves. We can *energetically* build healthy beautiful bodies and nourish our spirit by understanding how energy works within us and how we can work with our energy.

My Bodybrushing technique actually covers all seven energy centers, so as you're brushing, toweling and rubbing the oils into your body, you consciously draw attention to these centers. Try to envision the color and physical issue or relationship that the energy center has to your emotional and physical health.

I really feel centered when I use this as my own personal path to purification and connection. But there are times when I just simply jump out of bed and do my four-step program without the energy center connection. A lot of it depends on the time factor and the environment I'm in.

It's this simple: When your energy centers are out of whack, it manifests in your physical body as disease (or ill ease). Most of the time, our energy centers are out of balance because we are not aligned with our true spirit. We are not living our own personal truth. Each and every one of us is on a personal journey, and there are as many truths as there are people on the planet. My purpose here is to simply show you a purely beautiful way to love yourself and physically connect with your body, your energy centers and your spirit so you can draw on your awesome healing power within and live closer to your true spirit.

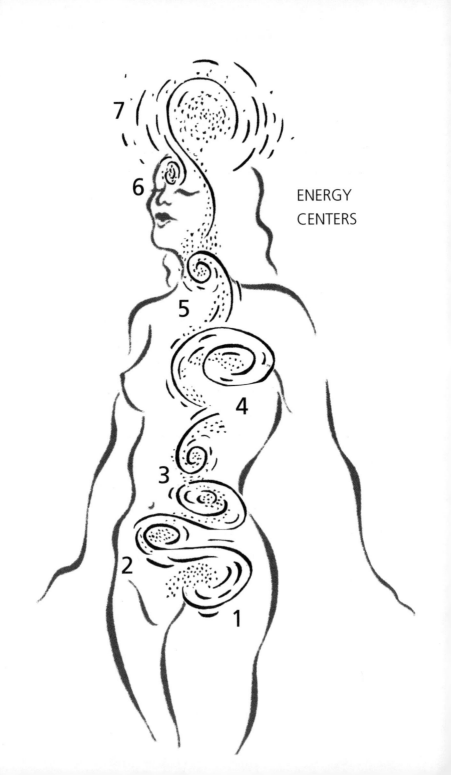

ENERGY
CENTERS

What follows is a brief explanation of your energy centers, their locations in your body, and their relationship to your organs and to various emotional and psychological issues as well as to the physical functions and dysfunction of your body. Use this, if you like, as your own personal ritual. Try it on and see if it fits. In order to demystify the Eastern terms used when talking about the body's energy centers, I will simply refer to them as energy center #1, #2, #3 and so forth.

Remember, when you body brush, you always begin with your toes and work your way up to the heart and head last. This pattern works perfectly because it allows you to begin connecting with your first energy center and it proceeds to the top of your head, ending with energy center #7, or the crown chakra.

ENERGY CENTER #1 (root/base) is the chakra at the base of the spine. Its center is physical energy and vitality. This energy center is our connection to traditional and familial beliefs. It is linked to the testicle and ovarian glands. You can stimulate this energy center while doing your morning Bodybrushing on any part of your body at or below the base of the spine. Visualize the color red when you are brushing, toweling or putting oil on your body in this area. Think of a family relationship that may need healing.

ENERGY CENTER #2 (sacral) is located a few inches above the base of the spine. Its center is desire, emotions, creativity, relationships and sexuality. It is linked to the adrenal glands. You can stimulate this energy center by visualizing the color orange while brushing, toweling or rubbing oils onto the abdomen, torso and buttocks. Think of doing one thing today that will get you closer to completing a goal.

ENERGY CENTER #3 (solar plexus) is located on the spine behind the navel. Its center is personal power and vitality, relationship and understanding of self. It is linked to the pancreas. This energy center can be stimulated by breathing deeply and bringing energy into the solar plexus area while performing brushing, toweling or oiling manipulations on this part of the body. Imagine yellow here. Think of loving, respecting and being honest with yourself today.

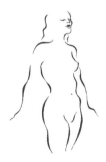

G l o w   T i p
Use Bodybrushing as the vehicle to learn
about your energy centers.

ENERGY CENTER #4 (heart) is located on the spine
behind the chest. This fourth center is the power center of
the human energy system. Its center is compassion and love.
It is linked to the thymus gland. You can stimulate this chakra
by concentrating on your heart pulsating, breathing in and
out deeply while brushing, toweling or rubbing your upper
torso and chest area. Picture the healthy color green in this
part of your body. Think of a relationship—friend or partner—in your life that needs healing.

ENERGY CENTER #5 (throat)
is located on the spine behind the
throat. It is linked to the thyroid
gland and its center is communica-
tion and expression, self-knowledge
and personal authority. At this point in
your Bodybrushing you are brushing,
rubbing or toweling your neck and
base of your head. Picture the color
blue here. Think of refraining from
making any judgments about
yourself or others today.

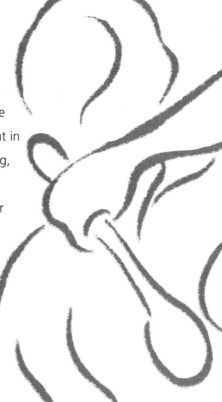

ENERGY CENTER #6 (brow or forehead) is the chakra of wisdom. It is located behind the space between the eyebrows and is linked to the pituitary gland. Its center is emotional intelligence and higher intuition. This energy center can be stimulated by visualizing the color indigo while brushing, toweling or rubbing this area. Think of drawing wisdom from your dreams.

ENERGY CENTER #7 (crown of the head) is located at the top of the head. It is the entry point for the human life-force and is linked to the brain's pineal gland. Its center is spirituality and enlightenment. It is concerned with spiritual balance and the relationship of the inner and outer selves. You can stimulate this energy center by visualizing a bright light. Think of performing a kind act for someone today.

Though somewhat wordy, the above ritual only takes a few moments to perform. Choose whichever part of the Body-brushing ritual you want and use it to connect with your energy centers. Work on connecting with one center a week until you become familiar with its power and purpose in your life. Soon you will be a master at locating blocked energy and connecting color, emotion and physical function with its relation to your own energy centers.

This practical application with your energy centers when you are fully awake rather than in a state of meditation is very stimulating. You are actually manually assisting your body in its quest to maintain health and spiritual balance. This is powerful "self-healthing."

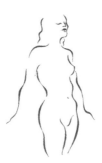 Use the energy chart on page *140* to help you become acquainted with the different energy centers, their corresponding colors and their relationship to your emotional and physical health. Once you begin this path to self-discovery, you will notice a whole new world of color and meaning opening up to you. You will become so much more aware of colors and their expression in nature, and you can constantly connect these colors with the corresponding energy centers of your body and what their physical and emotional significance are to you. It is unbelievably fascinating and joyous to heighten your awareness in this way.

G l o w   T i p
Get *Rhythms of the Chakras* CD and listen
to these tribal sounds as you manipulate
the oils into your skin.

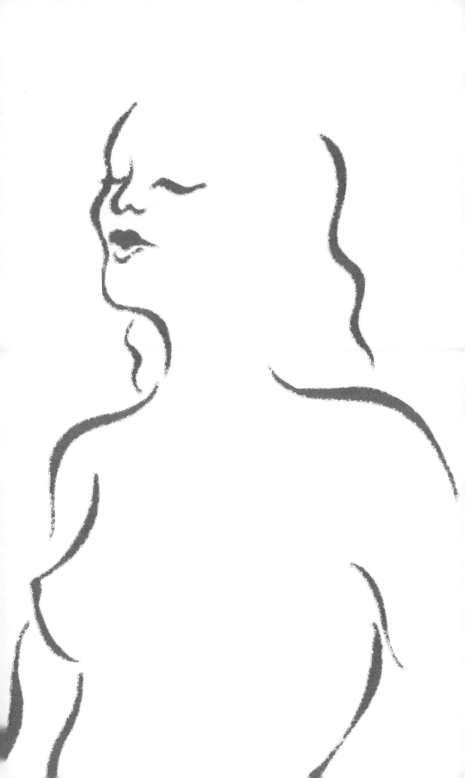

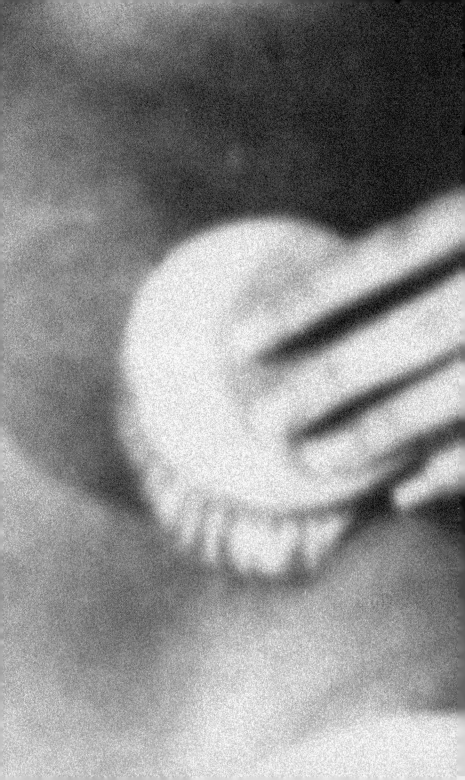

What's

Bodybrushing?

. . . And Other Frequently
Asked Questions

For one of my clients, Bodybrushing started out as a slightly eccentric, nerve-racking experience. She wondered, Was she brushing too hard? Too soft? Was she going in the right direction? Would she scratch her skin and would people think she was into some masochistic ritual? Let's dispel all doubts and answer some of these questions. FIRST . . .

What IS Bodybrushing?
Bodybrushing is the daily practice of using a natural vegetable bristle brush to exfoliate, clean your skin and stimulate your lymphatic system. Sometimes it is referred to as "dry brushing" because you do this before your bath when your skin is dry.

Where do I DO my Bodybrushing?
You can body brush anywhere you feel comfortable about being naked and performing this somewhat unusual but stimulating ritual. Most people do it in the privacy of their bathroom in front of their bathroom counter.

How long does Bodybrushing take?

It can take as little as five minutes, or you can spend longer when you have the time.

Can men do this too?

Are you kidding? Men were made for Bodybrushing. This is all about using a tool. And Bodybrushing is a fabulous tool.

Does Bodybrushing hurt or will it scratch my skin?

Goodness, no! If your skin is scratched or if it hurts, you are brushing too hard. Begin brushing lightly and increase the pressure as your skin becomes accustomed to it.

Are there any side effects to Bodybrushing?

Yes. And they are wonderful! A few of my clients *have* noticed a slight rash that lasts a day or two after the first couple of days of Bodybrushing. This is great because it means that toxins are leaving their body. You may notice increased perspiration due to the increased circulation and stimulation of your blood flow. This is good. Again, more toxins are leaving the body. Your body will regulate itself to this extra stimulation in a few weeks and you'll feel better than ever.

Can I overexfoliate my skin?

Yes, by using harsh chemicals and scrubs, but certainly not by
Bodybrushing regularly.

What happens to all my skin cells?

Over one million cells a day are shed from your skin. Ninety
percent of household dust is skin cells. Most of the cells you
shed from Bodybrushing will accumulate in your brushes, so
they need to be cleaned every so often.

Is it okay to brush my face?

Yes. You can brush your face very lightly with a soft facial brush.

Can I brush my face if I have acne?

You don't want to brush any part of your body that has
a skin irritation.

Will my skin be more sun sensitive?

No, but you must always protect your skin from the sun's
harmful rays. Use sunblock or simply cover yourself with
clothing or stay in the shade.

Do the seasons affect the type of oil I should use?

No. The recipe for oil in this book is good for any time of year.

Can I overstimulate my lymphatic system?

No. Stimulating your lymphatic system increases your white blood cell count. You can never have too strong an immune system.

What if I can't reach my back to body brush?

Enlist the help of your mate or a family member—or be satisfied that you have brushed and stimulated 95 percent of your body.

Can I body brush just once a week or do I have to do it every day?

You can do it once a week, but you'll probably end up doing it every day because you'll become addicted to how good you feel when you body brush. You'll simply have to perform this loving ritual on your body every day.

Is it all right if my friends and family use my brushes too?

No, no, no! That's forbidden. You should come to cherish your tools and covet them as your very own. Do you really want their skin cells on your brushes?

How do I clean my brushes?

That's easy. Once or twice a month, clean them with soap and warm water. Rinse well and let them air dry— in the sun, if possible.

When should I replace my brushes?

After you wash them a few times, you may notice the bristles become softer. Replace them when you feel they are no longer firm enough for you. I replace mine two or three times a year.

What about loofahs and sponges? Do they work the same as brushes?

No. Skin brushing is done dry. Loofahs and sponges are used in the shower when your skin is wet. It is an altogether different technique.

Can I use the brush on wet skin? Will it have the same effect?

No. When your skin is wet, it is much more sensitive to brushing and rubbing. It may cause sagging.

Do I have to give up soap and hot water?

Remember, your skin gets CLEAN from Bodybrushing. If you can't give up hot water, limit your time in the hot water to a few seconds and alternate with cold bursts of water. Use soap sparingly on the parts of your body you want to wash every day.

Will using one application of oil on my body as a moisturizer be enough?

Yes, definitely. The rich vitamin-packed plant oil is super skin food that outperforms any of those chemical-laden goos. It's a myth that you must apply lotion all day long to keep your skin moisturized. Even more importantly, Bodybrushing stimulates the oil-producing glands and boosts the body's own moisturizing process.

Won't the oil get all over my clothes and bedding?

When you apply oil lightly and manipulate it into your skin, you will only experience luxurious velvety-feeling skin. There will be no residue.

Will Bodybrushing REALLY make me feel younger and look better?

Absolutely. You will immediately know what I mean by GLOW!

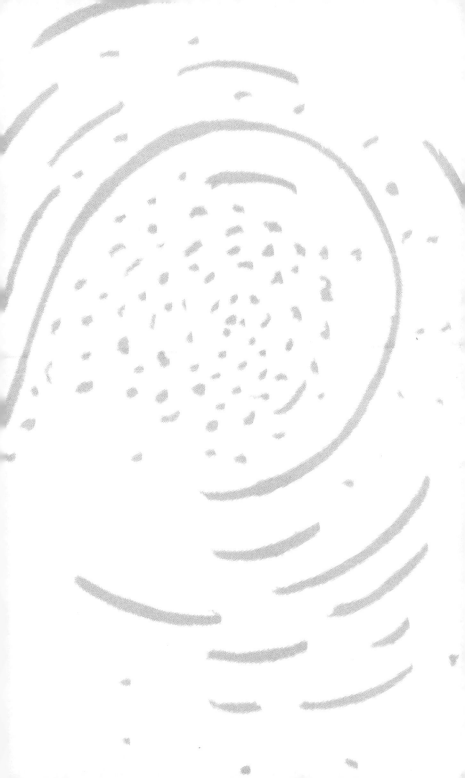

afterglow

What do my clients tell me now?

We don't need you anymore, Donna!

After a few months of Bodybrushing and a few body oil renewals, my clients no longer require my assistance or support. They are making their own body oils and using their energy charts with self-confidence. They are completely independent of product hype and enjoying the freedom of knowing how to maintain beautiful, healthy skin on their own.

I recently called on a number of my clients to ask them this important question: *What does your Bodybrushing program mean to you?* The responses were wonderfully similar:

~ IT'S THE ONLY WAY I WOULD EVER CONSIDER
   TAKING CARE OF MY SKIN.

~ SOMETHING WOULD BE MISSING IF I DIDN'T
   PERFORM MY DAILY BRUSHING RITUAL.

~ I DON'T FEEL CLEAN IF I DON'T PERFORM THIS
   SYSTEM EVERY DAY.

~ IT'S THE BEST HEALTH TOOL I'VE EVER USED.

~ I WOULDN'T DREAM OF CARING FOR MYSELF
   ANY OTHER WAY.

These words are joy to my ears. My dream to change the way the world wakes up is coming true. Every individual who performs this loving ritual is one more person on the planet who is getting a healthier lymphatic system, fostering a connection within, and maintaining radiant, gorgeous skin.

Reveal Your Glow: Brush Your Body Beautiful evolved from my personal journey toward self-discovery. One begins such a journey by embracing programs or systems like "GLOW" and committing to the nurturing of our mind and soul. Bodybrushing, I know, can be your vehicle to this "glow" that starts from within and ultimately radiates from your healthy, vibrant skin.

I am honored to be a part of your journey to health and beauty.

Celebrate yourself each and every day by Bodybrushing!

Joyfully yours,

Donna Rae

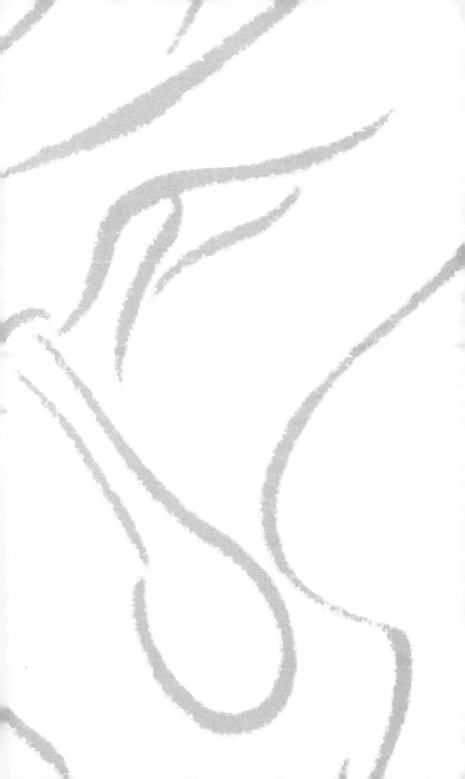

A p p e n d i x

REFERENCES AND RECOMMENDED READING

Anatomy of the Spirit by Caroline Myss (New York: Three Rivers Press, 1996).

Ancient Secret of the Fountain of Youth by Peter Kelder (New York: Doubleday, 1998).

Are You Confused? by Dr. Paavo Airola (Sherwood, OR: Health Plus Publishers, 1971).

The Art of the Bath by Sara Slavin and Karl Petzke (San Francisco, CA: Chronicle Books, 1997).

Don't Go to the Cosmetics Counter Without Me by Paula Begoun (Seattle, WA: Beginning Press, 1996).

Encyclopedia of Anti-Aging Remedies by John Heinerman, Ph.D. (Paramus, NJ: Prentice Hall, 1997).

The Gift of Touch by Helen Colton (New York: Kensington Books, 1983).

How to Live Longer and Feel Better by Linus Pauling (New York: Avon Books, 1987).

Is Your Body Trying to Tell You Something? by Carmen Renee Barry (Berkeley, CA: PageMill Press, 1997).

Joni Loughran's Natural Skin Care: Alternative & Traditional Techniques by Joni Loughran (Berkeley, CA: Frog Ltd. Books, 1996).

Kathryn Marsden's Super Skin by Kathryn Marsden (Great Britain: Thorsons, 1993).

Natural Organic Hair and Skin Care by Aubrey Hampton (Tampa, FL: Organica Press, 1987).

The Secret Language of the Soul by Jane Hope (San Francisco, CA: Chronicle Books, 1997).

The Seven Spiritual Laws of Success by Deepak Chopra (San Rafael, CA, and Novato, CA: Amber-Allen Publishing and New World Library, 1994).

The Skin Care Book: Simple Herbal Recipes by Kathlyn
Quatrochi (Loveland, CO: Interweave Press, Inc., 1997).

Vitamin Guide: Essential Nutrients for Healthy Living by
Hasnain Walji (Rockport, MA: Element Books, Inc., 1992).

*Wheels of Light: Chakras, Auras, and the Healing Energy of
the Body* by Rosalyn L. Bruyere (New York: Fireside/Simon &
Schuster, 1989).

Yoga: The Spirit and Practice of Moving into Stillness by Erich
Schiffmann (New York: Pocket Books/Simon & Schuster,
1996).

PRODUCT RESOURCES

My GLOW kit contains all the tools you need to get started with my Bodybrushing program. It has three natural fiber brushes, one coarse terry cloth, "Bufferi" towel, four ounces of pure plant and vitamin oil and a 15-minute instructional video. Use the order form in this book to get your very own GLOW Kit!

If you are an independent hunter-gatherer and want to get the tools on your own, the following resources are available.

Brushes

Hair Doc Company
16870 Stagg Street
Van Nuys, CA 91406
Tel: (818) 989-4247
Fax: (818) 989-1156
To order, call for a VNS Nutrition catalog: (800) 681-7099

Yerba Prima
740 Jefferson Avenue
Ashland, OR 97520-3743
Tel: (800) 488-4339
Fax: (541) 488-2443
e-mail: yerba@yerba.com

Harry D. Koenig & Co., Inc.

7 Main Street

East Rockaway, NY 11518

Tel: (516) 599-1776

Fax: (516) 599-1451

$85.00 minimum order. Call for catalog.

Towels

You can find coarse terry
towels at discount ware-
house stores like
Costco or Wal Mart,
or try Kmart Stores.
Call for a Kmart
store near you:
(800) 63-KMART

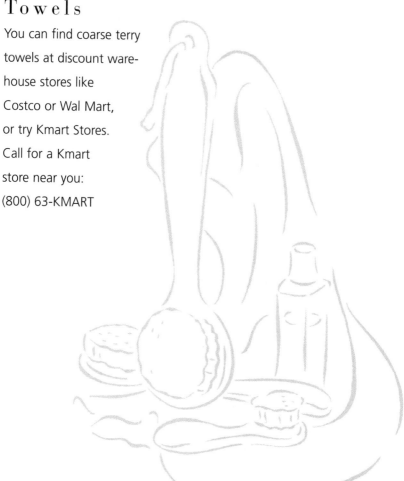

Oils

If you want to mix your own oils as discussed in chapter 7
of this book, you can buy pure plant oils at your local health
food store. Again, avocado oil is the very best base oil you can
use. If you can't find it easily, use apricot kernel oil. Olive oil is
also wonderful, but a bit pungent. You can also mail order
from the following:

Aura Cacia
101 Paymaster Road
Weaverville, CA 96093
Tel: (800) 437-3301
Fax: (319) 227-7966
Web site: www.auracacia.com

Vitamins

I use gel capsules in combination with the above oils. You can
find evening primrose, vitamins A, D and E at your local health
food store. Or contact the following:

General Nutrition Center (GNC)
Call for a GNC store near you: (800) 477-4462

Or go to your local health food store and check for the
vitamins you need there.

Order form

Phone Orders: Toll FREE 1-877-YOU-GLOW or 1- 800-749-0029
Online Orders: www.bodyshine.com
Postal Orders: EarthTime Publications, 1324 State Street, Suite J292
Santa Barbara, CA 93101

Please send me _____ copies of *Reveal Your Glow: Brush Your Body Beautiful*
@ $14.95 each

Please send me _____ copies of the 15-minute instructional Bodybrushing video
@ $10.95 each

I WANT TO GET GLOWING NOW!

Please send me _____ GLOW Kits made by BodyShine™ @ $59.95 each
(Includes three brushes, one "Bufferi" towel, four ounces of pure plant oil and
15-minute Bodybrushing instructional video)

You can reorder individual items from the GLOW Kit. Call the toll-free number
for more information.

Please add 7.75% for books and kits shipped to California addresses.

SHIPPING:
$4.00 for the first book and $2.00 for each additional book. $6.00 for the
first kit and $4.00 for each additional kit.

Subtotal $ _____
Tax. CA addresses add 7.75% $ _____
Shipping $ _____
TOTAL $ _____

Make checks payable to: EarthTime Publications

❑ Check   ❑ VISA   ❑ MasterCard   ❑ Discover

SHIP TO:

Name:_____

Address:_____

City:_____State:_____Zip:_____

Phone:_____E:mail:_____

Card number: _____

Name on card: _____ Exp. date: _____/_____

Signature of cardholder: _____

About the Author

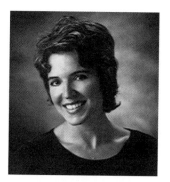

Donna Rae has been in the
health and beauty industry for
over 15 years. She has studied
cosmetology, herbology and
naturopathy as well as business
and finance. In recent years,
teaching people how to GLOW using her Bodybrushing
technique has become Donna's passion and profession.

Raised on ranches in Oregon and Washington state, Rae has
been guided by the healing powers of nature and has taken
the path of natural beauty since childhood.

Donna Rae is currently writing her second and third books
entitled *Revealing Rituals* and *A Million Masks of Mother.* She
lives with her family in Santa Barbara.

Donna Rae would like to hear from you. If *Reveal Your Glow*
has led you to a healthier lifestyle, please write to:

Donna Rae, 1324 State Street, Suite J292
Santa Barbara, California 93101

Donna Rae is available for lectures, seminars, guest
appearances and private consultation. Details will be
sent upon request.